NP
H&P

For More NP Clinical Products visit:
www.renursingedu.com

This page is intentionally left blank

Date:	Initials/MRN:	Age:	Rotation:

CC: _____ y/o M/F
HPI: *symptoms/pertinent +/- ROS/prior episodes/recent travel/sick contacts*

PMHx *child/adult illness /hospitalizations/ immunizations*

SurgHx *type/when/ why/complications*

FamHx *parents/siblings/ children*

SHx *smoker/ETOH/illicits/exercise/sex/maritalstatus*

Allergies *meds/foods/ environmental/reactions*

Meds *reason/dose/time/route/compliance/vitamins/ herbs/otcs*

ROS (circle any)

Gen
Fatigue
Weight +/-
Chills
Night sweats
Eyes
Pain
Redness
Vision changes
ENT
Headache
Hoarseness
Sore throat
Sinus sx
Hearing loss
Tinnitus
Runny nose

Pulm
Cough
SOB
Wheezing
Hemoptysis
CV
Chest pain
Edema
PND
Orthopnea
Palpitations
Claudication
GI
Abd pain
N/V
Heartburn
Bloody stools

GU
Dysuria
Frequency
Hematuria
Discharge
Flank pain
MS
Arthralgia
Arthritis
Joint swelling
Myalgias
Back pain
Heme
Bleeding
Bruising
Lymph
Swelling

Endo
Polyuria
Polydypsia
Polyphagia
Derm
Rash
Pruritis
Wound(s)
Neuro
Weakness
Seizures
Parasthesias
Tremors
Syncope
Psych
Anxiety
Depression

+ ROS Findings

PE vitals   HR   BP   RR   T   SPO2   Ht   Wt   BMI%

(check any)	**Neck**	**Pulm**	**Neuro**
General	( ) Midline trachea	( ) No retractions	( ) AAO x 3
( ) No Acute Distress	( ) nl thyroid w/o	( ) No dullness	( ) CN II-XII intact
( ) Cooperative	enlargement	( ) No fremitus	( ) nl sensation
( ) nl Hygiene	( ) No	( ) No wheezing/	( ) Reflexes 2+ &
Eyes	lymphadenopathy	rales/rhonchi	symmetrical
( ) nl conjunctiva	**CV**	**GI**	( ) nl memory
( ) PERRLA	( ) PMI	( ) No masses/	( ) nl speech
( ) Size___	nondisplaced	tenderness	**MSK**
( ) nl Fundus	( ) No murmur/	( ) No hep/	( ) nl tone
( ) nl Discs/vessels	gallop/rub	splenomegaly	( ) nl bulk
( ) No scleral icterus	( ) nl intensity w/o	( ) nl bowel sounds	( ) nl gait
ENT	bruit	( ) No dullness	( ) nl ROM UE
( ) No scars/masses	( ) No JVD	( ) Heme (-) stool	( ) nl ROM LE
( ) nl canals/ TM	( ) nl femoral/pedal	**GU**	L___/5 UE R___/5
( ) nl hearing bilat	pulses	( ) nl ext genitalia	L___/5 LE R___/5
( ) nl teeth/tongue	( ) No pedal	( ) No hernia	
	edema		

+ PE Findings

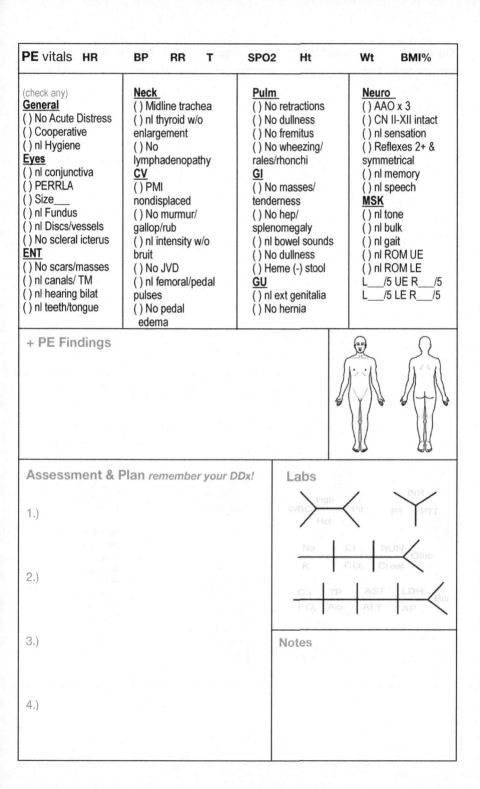

Assessment & Plan *remember your DDx!*

1.)

2.)

3.)

4.)

Labs

Hgb
WBC   Plt
Hct

INR
PT   PTT

Na   Cl   BUN
                          Gluc
K   CO₂   Creat

Ca   TP   AST   LDH
                          Bili
PO₄   Alb   ALT   AP

Notes

| **Date:** | **Initials/MRN:** | **Age:** | **Rotation:** |

CC: _____ y/o M/F
HPI: *symptoms/pertinent +/- ROS/prior episodes/recent travel/sick contacts*

| **PMHx** *child/adult illness /hospitalizations/ immunizations* | **SurgHx** *type/when/ why/complications* | **FamHx** *parents/siblings/ children* |

SHx *smoker/ETOH/illicits/exercise/sex/maritalstatus*

| **Allergies** *meds/foods/ environmental/reactions* | **Meds** *reason/dose/time/route/compliance/vitamins/ herbs/otcs* |

ROS (circle any)

Gen	**Pulm**	**GU**	**Endo**
Fatigue	Cough	Dysuria	Polyuria
Weight +/-	SOB	Frequency	Polydypsia
Chills	Wheezing	Hematuria	Polyphagia
Night sweats	Hemoptysis	Discharge	**Derm**
Eyes	**CV**	Flank pain	Rash
Pain	Chest pain	**MS**	Pruritis
Redness	Edema	Arthralgia	Wound(s)
Vision changes	PND	Arthritis	**Neuro**
ENT	Orthopnea	Joint swelling	Weakness
Headache	Palpitations	Myalgias	Seizures
Hoarseness	Claudication	Back pain	Parasthesias
Sore throat	**GI**	**Heme**	Tremors
Sinus sx	Abd pain	Bleeding	Syncope
Hearing loss	N/V	Bruising	**Psych**
Tinnitus	Heartburn	**Lymph**	Anxiety
Runny nose	Bloody stools	Swelling	Depression

+ ROS Findings

PE vitals HR   BP   RR   T   SPO2   Ht   Wt   BMI%

(check any)	**Neck**	**Pulm**	**Neuro**
General	( ) Midline trachea	( ) No retractions	( ) AAO x 3
( ) No Acute Distress	( ) nl thyroid w/o	( ) No dullness	( ) CN II-XII intact
( ) Cooperative	enlargement	( ) No fremitus	( ) nl sensation
( ) nl Hygiene	( ) No	( ) No wheezing/	( ) Reflexes 2+ &
Eyes	lymphadenopathy	rales/rhonchi	symmetrical
( ) nl conjunctiva	**CV**	**GI**	( ) nl memory
( ) PERRLA	( ) PMI	( ) No masses/	( ) nl speech
( ) Size___	nondisplaced	tenderness	**MSK**
( ) nl Fundus	( ) No murmur/	( ) No hep/	( ) nl tone
( ) nl Discs/vessels	gallop/rub	splenomegaly	( ) nl bulk
( ) No scleral icterus	( ) nl intensity w/o	( ) nl bowel sounds	( ) nl gait
ENT	bruit	( ) No dullness	( ) nl ROM UE
( ) No scars/masses	( ) No JVD	( ) Heme (-) stool	( ) nl ROM LE
( ) nl canals/ TM	( ) nl femoral/pedal	**GU**	L___/5 UE R___/5
( ) nl hearing bilat	pulses	( ) nl ext genitalia	L___/5 LE R___/5
( ) nl teeth/tongue	( ) No pedal	( ) No hernia	
	edema		

+ PE Findings

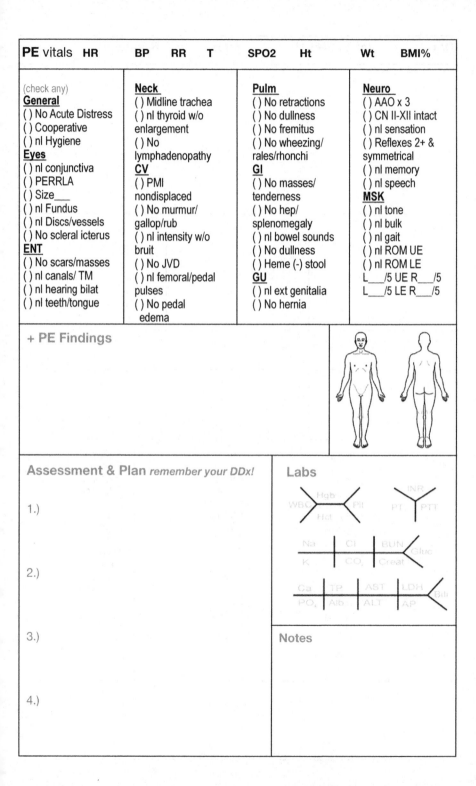

Assessment & Plan *remember your DDx!*

1.)

2.)

3.)

4.)

Labs

Notes

Date:	Initials/MRN:	Age:	Rotation:

CC: _____ y/o M/F
HPI: *symptoms/pertinent +/- ROS/prior episodes/recent travel/sick contacts*

PMHx *child/adult illness /hospitalizations/ immunizations*

SurgHx *type/when/ why/complications*

FamHx *parents/siblings/ children*

SHx *smoker/ETOH/illicits/exercise/sex/maritalstatus*

Allergies *meds/foods/ environmental/reactions*

Meds *reason/dose/time/route/compliance/vitamins/ herbs/otcs*

ROS (circle any)

Gen
Fatigue
Weight +/-
Chills
Night sweats
Eyes
Pain
Redness
Vision changes
ENT
Headache
Hoarseness
Sore throat
Sinus sx
Hearing loss
Tinnitus
Runny nose

Pulm
Cough
SOB
Wheezing
Hemoptysis
CV
Chest pain
Edema
PND
Orthopnea
Palpitations
Claudication
GI
Abd pain
N/V
Heartburn
Bloody stools

GU
Dysuria
Frequency
Hematuria
Discharge
Flank pain
MS
Arthralgia
Arthritis
Joint swelling
Myalgias
Back pain
Heme
Bleeding
Bruising
Lymph
Swelling

Endo
Polyuria
Polydypsia
Polyphagia
Derm
Rash
Pruritis
Wound(s)
Neuro
Weakness
Seizures
Parasthesias
Tremors
Syncope
Psych
Anxiety
Depression

+ ROS Findings

PE vitals   **HR**   **BP**   **RR**   **T**   **SPO2**   **Ht**   **Wt**   **BMI%**

(check any)

General
( ) No Acute Distress
( ) Cooperative
( ) nl Hygiene
Eyes
( ) nl conjunctiva
( ) PERRLA
( ) Size___
( ) nl Fundus
( ) nl Discs/vessels
( ) No scleral icterus
ENT
( ) No scars/masses
( ) nl canals/ TM
( ) nl hearing bilat
( ) nl teeth/tongue

Neck
( ) Midline trachea
( ) nl thyroid w/o
enlargement
( ) No
lymphadenopathy
CV
( ) PMI
nondisplaced
( ) No murmur/
gallop/rub
( ) nl intensity w/o
bruit
( ) No JVD
( ) nl femoral/pedal
pulses
( ) No pedal
edema

Pulm
( ) No retractions
( ) No dullness
( ) No fremitus
( ) No wheezing/
rales/rhonchi
GI
( ) No masses/
tenderness
( ) No hep/
splenomegaly
( ) nl bowel sounds
( ) No dullness
( ) Heme (-) stool
GU
( ) nl ext genitalia
( ) No hernia

Neuro
( ) AAO x 3
( ) CN II-XII intact
( ) nl sensation
( ) Reflexes 2+ &
symmetrical
( ) nl memory
( ) nl speech
MSK
( ) nl tone
( ) nl bulk
( ) nl gait
( ) nl ROM UE
( ) nl ROM LE
L___/5 UE R___/5
L___/5 LE R___/5

+ PE Findings

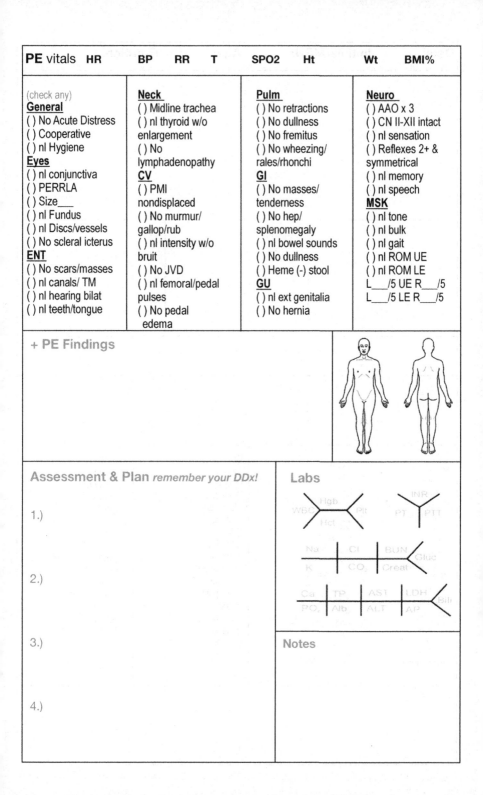

Assessment & Plan *remember your DDx!*

1.)

2.)

3.)

4.)

Labs

Notes

Date:	**Initials/MRN:**	**Age:**	**Rotation:**

CC: _____ y/o M/F
HPI: *symptoms/pertinent +/- ROS/prior episodes/recent travel/sick contacts*

PMHx *child/adult illness /hospitalizations/ immunizations*	**SurgHx** *type/when/ why/complications*	**FamHx** *parents/siblings/ children*

SHx *smoker/ETOH/illicits/exercise/sex/maritalstatus*

Allergies *meds/foods/ environmental/reactions*	**Meds** *reason/dose/time/route/compliance/vitamins/ herbs/otcs*

ROS (circle any)

Gen	**Pulm**	**GU**	**Endo**
Fatigue	Cough	Dysuria	Polyuria
Weight +/-	SOB	Frequency	Polydypsia
Chills	Wheezing	Hematuria	Polyphagia
Night sweats	Hemoptysis	Discharge	**Derm**
Eyes	**CV**	Flank pain	Rash
Pain	Chest pain	**MS**	Pruritis
Redness	Edema	Arthralgia	Wound(s)
Vision changes	PND	Arthritis	**Neuro**
ENT	Orthopnea	Joint swelling	Weakness
Headache	Palpitations	Myalgias	Seizures
Hoarseness	Claudication	Back pain	Parasthesias
Sore throat	**GI**	**Heme**	Tremors
Sinus sx	Abd pain	Bleeding	Syncope
Hearing loss	N/V	Bruising	**Psych**
Tinnitus	Heartburn	**Lymph**	Anxiety
Runny nose	Bloody stools	Swelling	Depression

+ ROS Findings

PE vitals   **HR**   **BP**   **RR**   **T**   **SPO2**   **Ht**   **Wt**   **BMI%**

(check any) **General**	**Neck**	**Pulm**	**Neuro**
( ) No Acute Distress	( ) Midline trachea	( ) No retractions	( ) AAO x 3
( ) Cooperative	( ) nl thyroid w/o	( ) No dullness	( ) CN II-XII intact
( ) nl Hygiene	enlargement	( ) No fremitus	( ) nl sensation
Eyes	( ) No	( ) No wheezing/	( ) Reflexes 2+ &
( ) nl conjunctiva	lymphadenopathy	rales/rhonchi	symmetrical
( ) PERRLA	**CV**	**GI**	( ) nl memory
( ) Size___	( ) PMI	( ) No masses/	( ) nl speech
( ) nl Fundus	nondisplaced	tenderness	**MSK**
( ) nl Discs/vessels	( ) No murmur/	( ) No hep/	( ) nl tone
( ) No scleral icterus	gallop/rub	splenomegaly	( ) nl bulk
ENT	( ) nl intensity w/o	( ) nl bowel sounds	( ) nl gait
( ) No scars/masses	bruit	( ) No dullness	( ) nl ROM UE
( ) nl canals/ TM	( ) No JVD	( ) Heme (-) stool	( ) nl ROM LE
( ) nl hearing bilat	( ) nl femoral/pedal	**GU**	L___/5 UE R___/5
( ) nl teeth/tongue	pulses	( ) nl ext genitalia	L___/5 LE R___/5
	( ) No pedal	( ) No hernia	
	edema		

+ PE Findings

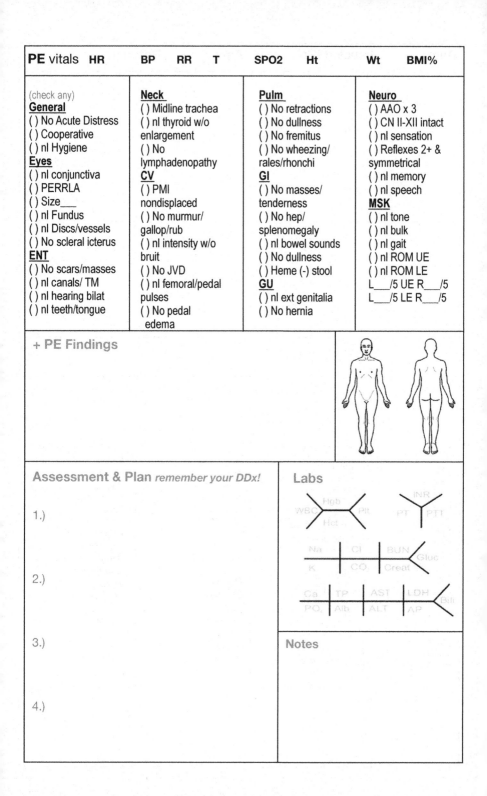

Assessment & Plan *remember your DDx!*

1.)

2.)

3.)

4.)

Labs

Notes

Date:	Initials/MRN:	Age:	Rotation:

CC: _____ y/o M/F
HPI: *symptoms/pertinent +/- ROS/prior episodes/recent travel/sick contacts*

PMHx *child/adult illness /hospitalizations/ immunizations*

SurgHx *type/when/ why/complications*

FamHx *parents/siblings/ children*

SHx *smoker/ETOH/illicits/exercise/sex/maritalstatus*

Allergies *meds/foods/ environmental/reactions*

Meds *reason/dose/time/route/compliance/vitamins/ herbs/otcs*

ROS (circle any)

Gen
Fatigue
Weight +/-
Chills
Night sweats
Eyes
Pain
Redness
Vision changes
ENT
Headache
Hoarseness
Sore throat
Sinus sx
Hearing loss
Tinnitus
Runny nose

Pulm
Cough
SOB
Wheezing
Hemoptysis
CV
Chest pain
Edema
PND
Orthopnea
Palpitations
Claudication
GI
Abd pain
N/V
Heartburn
Bloody stools

GU
Dysuria
Frequency
Hematuria
Discharge
Flank pain
MS
Arthralgia
Arthritis
Joint swelling
Myalgias
Back pain
Heme
Bleeding
Bruising
Lymph
Swelling

Endo
Polyuria
Polydypsia
Polyphagia
Derm
Rash
Pruritis
Wound(s)
Neuro
Weakness
Seizures
Parasthesias
Tremors
Syncope
Psych
Anxiety
Depression

+ ROS Findings

PE vitals	HR	BP	RR	T	SPO2	Ht		Wt	BMI%

(check any) **General**	**Neck**	**Pulm**	**Neuro**
( ) No Acute Distress	( ) Midline trachea	( ) No retractions	( ) AAO x 3
( ) Cooperative	( ) nl thyroid w/o	( ) No dullness	( ) CN II-XII intact
( ) nl Hygiene	enlargement	( ) No fremitus	( ) nl sensation
Eyes	( ) No	( ) No wheezing/	( ) Reflexes 2+ &
( ) nl conjunctiva	lymphadenopathy	rales/rhonchi	symmetrical
( ) PERRLA	**CV**	**GI**	( ) nl memory
( ) Size___	( ) PMI	( ) No masses/	( ) nl speech
( ) nl Fundus	nondisplaced	tenderness	**MSK**
( ) nl Discs/vessels	( ) No murmur/	( ) No hep/	( ) nl tone
( ) No scleral icterus	gallop/rub	splenomegaly	( ) nl bulk
ENT	( ) nl intensity w/o	( ) nl bowel sounds	( ) nl gait
( ) No scars/masses	bruit	( ) No dullness	( ) nl ROM UE
( ) nl canals/ TM	( ) No JVD	( ) Heme (-) stool	( ) nl ROM LE
( ) nl hearing bilat	( ) nl femoral/pedal	**GU**	L___/5 UE R___/5
( ) nl teeth/tongue	pulses	( ) nl ext genitalia	L___/5 LE R___/5
	( ) No pedal	( ) No hernia	
	edema		

+ PE Findings

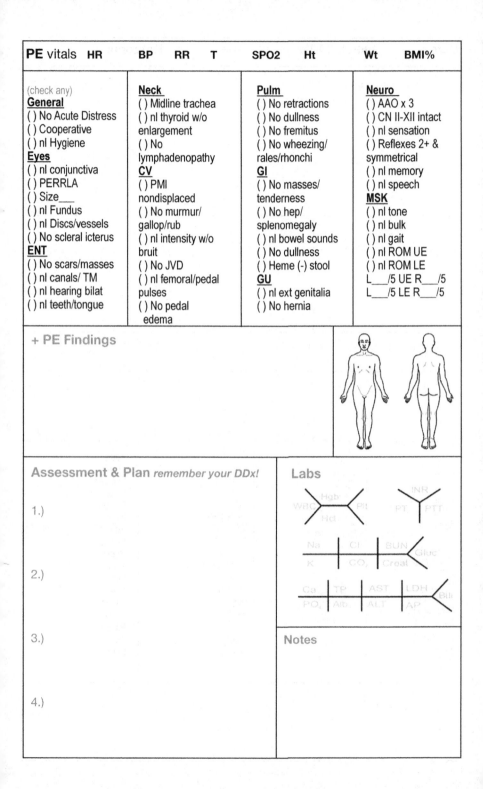

Assessment & Plan *remember your DDx!*

1.)

2.)

3.)

4.)

Labs

Notes

| Date: | Initials/MRN: | Age: | Rotation: |

CC: _____ y/o M/F
HPI: *symptoms/pertinent +/- ROS/prior episodes/recent travel/sick contacts*

| **PMHx** *child/adult illness /hospitalizations/ immunizations* | **SurgHx** *type/when/ why/complications* | **FamHx** *parents/siblings/ children* |

SHx *smoker/ETOH/illicits/exercise/sex/maritalstatus*

| **Allergies** *meds/foods/ environmental/reactions* | **Meds** *reason/dose/time/route/compliance/vitamins/ herbs/otcs* |

ROS (circle any)

Gen	**Pulm**	**GU**	**Endo**
Fatigue	Cough	Dysuria	Polyuria
Weight +/-	SOB	Frequency	Polydypsia
Chills	Wheezing	Hematuria	Polyphagia
Night sweats	Hemoptysis	Discharge	**Derm**
Eyes	**CV**	Flank pain	Rash
Pain	Chest pain	**MS**	Pruritis
Redness	Edema	Arthralgia	Wound(s)
Vision changes	PND	Arthritis	**Neuro**
ENT	Orthopnea	Joint swelling	Weakness
Headache	Palpitations	Myalgias	Seizures
Hoarseness	Claudication	Back pain	Parasthesias
Sore throat	**GI**	**Heme**	Tremors
Sinus sx	Abd pain	Bleeding	Syncope
Hearing loss	N/V	Bruising	**Psych**
Tinnitus	Heartburn	**Lymph**	Anxiety
Runny nose	Bloody stools	Swelling	Depression

+ ROS Findings

PE vitals	**HR**	**BP**	**RR**	**T**	**SPO2**	**Ht**	**Wt**	**BMI%**

(check any)	**Neck**	**Pulm**	**Neuro**
General	( ) Midline trachea	( ) No retractions	( ) AAO x 3
( ) No Acute Distress	( ) nl thyroid w/o	( ) No dullness	( ) CN II-XII intact
( ) Cooperative	enlargement	( ) No fremitus	( ) nl sensation
( ) nl Hygiene	( ) No	( ) No wheezing/	( ) Reflexes 2+ &
Eyes	lymphadenopathy	rales/rhonchi	symmetrical
( ) nl conjunctiva	**CV**	**GI**	( ) nl memory
( ) PERRLA	( ) PMI	( ) No masses/	( ) nl speech
( ) Size___	nondisplaced	tenderness	**MSK**
( ) nl Fundus	( ) No murmur/	( ) No hep/	( ) nl tone
( ) nl Discs/vessels	gallop/rub	splenomegaly	( ) nl bulk
( ) No scleral icterus	( ) nl intensity w/o	( ) nl bowel sounds	( ) nl gait
ENT	bruit	( ) No dullness	( ) nl ROM UE
( ) No scars/masses	( ) No JVD	( ) Heme (-) stool	( ) nl ROM LE
( ) nl canals/ TM	( ) nl femoral/pedal	**GU**	L___/5 UE R___/5
( ) nl hearing bilat	pulses	( ) nl ext genitalia	L___/5 LE R___/5
( ) nl teeth/tongue	( ) No pedal	( ) No hernia	
	edema		

+ PE Findings

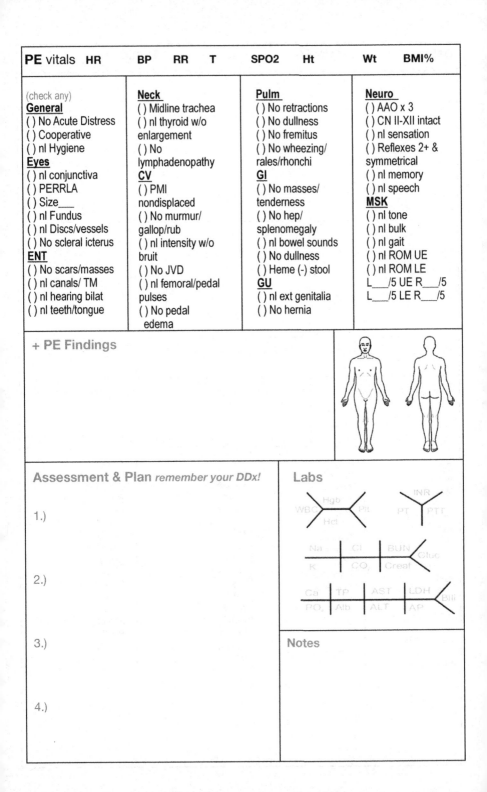

Assessment & Plan *remember your DDx!*

1.)

2.)

3.)

4.)

Labs

Notes

Date:	Initials/MRN:	Age:	Rotation:

CC: _____ y/o M/F
HPI: *symptoms/pertinent +/- ROS/prior episodes/recent travel/sick contacts*

PMHx *child/adult illness /hospitalizations/ immunizations*

SurgHx *type/when/ why/complications*

FamHx *parents/siblings/ children*

SHx *smoker/ETOH/illicits/exercise/sex/maritalstatus*

Allergies *meds/foods/ environmental/reactions*

Meds *reason/dose/time/route/compliance/vitamins/ herbs/otcs*

ROS (circle any)

Gen
Fatigue
Weight +/-
Chills
Night sweats
Eyes
Pain
Redness
Vision changes
ENT
Headache
Hoarseness
Sore throat
Sinus sx
Hearing loss
Tinnitus
Runny nose

Pulm
Cough
SOB
Wheezing
Hemoptysis
CV
Chest pain
Edema
PND
Orthopnea
Palpitations
Claudication
GI
Abd pain
N/V
Heartburn
Bloody stools

GU
Dysuria
Frequency
Hematuria
Discharge
Flank pain
MS
Arthralgia
Arthritis
Joint swelling
Myalgias
Back pain
Heme
Bleeding
Bruising
Lymph
Swelling

Endo
Polyuria
Polydypsia
Polyphagia
Derm
Rash
Pruritis
Wound(s)
Neuro
Weakness
Seizures
Parasthesias
Tremors
Syncope
Psych
Anxiety
Depression

+ ROS Findings

PE vitals	HR	BP	RR	T	SPO2	Ht	Wt	BMI%

(check any) **General** ( ) No Acute Distress ( ) Cooperative ( ) nl Hygiene **Eyes** ( ) nl conjunctiva ( ) PERRLA ( ) Size___ ( ) nl Fundus ( ) nl Discs/vessels ( ) No scleral icterus **ENT** ( ) No scars/masses ( ) nl canals/ TM ( ) nl hearing bilat ( ) nl teeth/tongue	**Neck** ( ) Midline trachea ( ) nl thyroid w/o enlargement ( ) No lymphadenopathy **CV** ( ) PMI nondisplaced ( ) No murmur/ gallop/rub ( ) nl intensity w/o bruit ( ) No JVD ( ) nl femoral/pedal pulses ( ) No pedal edema	**Pulm** ( ) No retractions ( ) No dullness ( ) No fremitus ( ) No wheezing/ rales/rhonchi **GI** ( ) No masses/ tenderness ( ) No hep/ splenomegaly ( ) nl bowel sounds ( ) No dullness ( ) Heme (-) stool **GU** ( ) nl ext genitalia ( ) No hernia	**Neuro** ( ) AAO x 3 ( ) CN II-XII intact ( ) nl sensation ( ) Reflexes 2+ & symmetrical ( ) nl memory ( ) nl speech **MSK** ( ) nl tone ( ) nl bulk ( ) nl gait ( ) nl ROM UE ( ) nl ROM LE L___/5 UE R___/5 L___/5 LE R___/5

+ PE Findings

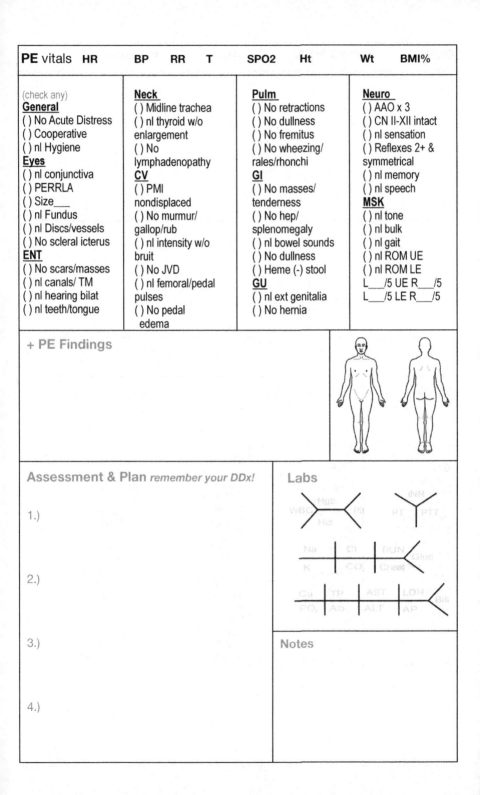

Assessment & Plan *remember your DDx!*

1.)

2.)

3.)

4.)

Labs

Notes

Date:	Initials/MRN:	Age:	Rotation:

CC: _____ y/o M/F

HPI: *symptoms/pertinent +/- ROS/prior episodes/recent travel/sick contacts*

PMHx *child/adult illness /hospitalizations/ immunizations*	**SurgHx** *type/when/ why/complications*	**FamHx** *parents/siblings/ children*

SHx *smoker/ETOH/illicits/exercise/sex/maritalstatus*

Allergies *meds/foods/ environmental/reactions*	**Meds** *reason/dose/time/route/compliance/vitamins/ herbs/otcs*

ROS (circle any)

Gen	**Pulm**	**GU**	**Endo**
Fatigue	Cough	Dysuria	Polyuria
Weight +/-	SOB	Frequency	Polydypsia
Chills	Wheezing	Hematuria	Polyphagia
Night sweats	Hemoptysis	Discharge	**Derm**
Eyes	**CV**	Flank pain	Rash
Pain	Chest pain	**MS**	Pruritis
Redness	Edema	Arthralgia	Wound(s)
Vision changes	PND	Arthritis	**Neuro**
ENT	Orthopnea	Joint swelling	Weakness
Headache	Palpitations	Myalgias	Seizures
Hoarseness	Claudication	Back pain	Parasthesias
Sore throat	**GI**	**Heme**	Tremors
Sinus sx	Abd pain	Bleeding	Syncope
Hearing loss	N/V	Bruising	**Psych**
Tinnitus	Heartburn	**Lymph**	Anxiety
Runny nose	Bloody stools	Swelling	Depression

+ ROS Findings

PE vitals   HR   BP   RR   T   SPO2   Ht   Wt   BMI%

(check any)	Neck	Pulm	Neuro
General	**Neck**	**Pulm**	**Neuro**
( ) No Acute Distress	( ) Midline trachea	( ) No retractions	( ) AAO x 3
( ) Cooperative	( ) nl thyroid w/o	( ) No dullness	( ) CN II-XII intact
( ) nl Hygiene	enlargement	( ) No fremitus	( ) nl sensation
Eyes	( ) No	( ) No wheezing/	( ) Reflexes 2+ &
( ) nl conjunctiva	lymphadenopathy	rales/rhonchi	symmetrical
( ) PERRLA	**CV**	**GI**	( ) nl memory
( ) Size___	( ) PMI	( ) No masses/	( ) nl speech
( ) nl Fundus	nondisplaced	tenderness	**MSK**
( ) nl Discs/vessels	( ) No murmur/	( ) No hep/	( ) nl tone
( ) No scleral icterus	gallop/rub	splenomegaly	( ) nl bulk
ENT	( ) nl intensity w/o	( ) nl bowel sounds	( ) nl gait
( ) No scars/masses	bruit	( ) No dullness	( ) nl ROM UE
( ) nl canals/ TM	( ) No JVD	( ) Heme (-) stool	( ) nl ROM LE
( ) nl hearing bilat	( ) nl femoral/pedal	**GU**	L___/5 UE R___/5
( ) nl teeth/tongue	pulses	( ) nl ext genitalia	L___/5 LE R___/5
	( ) No pedal	( ) No hernia	
	edema		

+ PE Findings

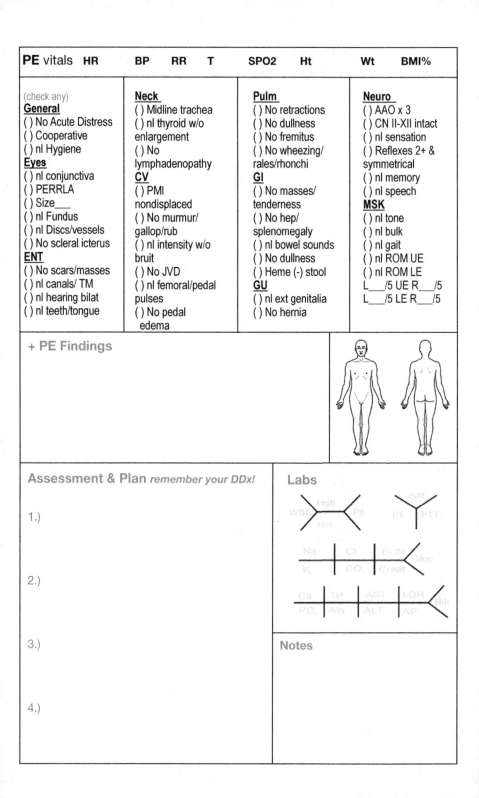

Assessment & Plan *remember your DDx!*

1.)

2.)

3.)

4.)

Labs

Hgb
WBC   Plt   INR
Hct   PT   PTT

Na   Cl   BUN
                         Gluc
K   CO₂   Creat

Ca   TP   AST   LDH
                              Bili
PO₄   Alb   ALT   AP

Notes

Date: **Initials/MRN:**   **Age:**   **Rotation:**

CC: _____ y/o M/F
HPI: *symptoms/pertinent +/- ROS/prior episodes/recent travel/sick contacts*

PMHx *child/adult illness /hospitalizations/ immunizations*

SurgHx *type/when/ why/complications*

FamHx *parents/siblings/ children*

SHx *smoker/ETOH/illicits/exercise/sex/maritalstatus*

Allergies *meds/foods/ environmental/reactions*

Meds *reason/dose/time/route/compliance/vitamins/ herbs/otcs*

ROS (circle any)

Gen
Fatigue
Weight +/-
Chills
Night sweats
Eyes
Pain
Redness
Vision changes
ENT
Headache
Hoarseness
Sore throat
Sinus sx
Hearing loss
Tinnitus
Runny nose

Pulm
Cough
SOB
Wheezing
Hemoptysis
CV
Chest pain
Edema
PND
Orthopnea
Palpitations
Claudication
GI
Abd pain
N/V
Heartburn
Bloody stools

GU
Dysuria
Frequency
Hematuria
Discharge
Flank pain
MS
Arthralgia
Arthritis
Joint swelling
Myalgias
Back pain
Heme
Bleeding
Bruising
Lymph
Swelling

Endo
Polyuria
Polydypsia
Polyphagia
Derm
Rash
Pruritis
Wound(s)
Neuro
Weakness
Seizures
Parasthesias
Tremors
Syncope
Psych
Anxiety
Depression

+ ROS Findings

PE vitals	HR	BP	RR	T	SPO2	Ht	Wt	BMI%

(check any) **General** ( ) No Acute Distress ( ) Cooperative ( ) nl Hygiene **Eyes** ( ) nl conjunctiva ( ) PERRLA ( ) Size___ ( ) nl Fundus ( ) nl Discs/vessels ( ) No scleral icterus **ENT** ( ) No scars/masses ( ) nl canals/ TM ( ) nl hearing bilat ( ) nl teeth/tongue	**Neck** ( ) Midline trachea ( ) nl thyroid w/o enlargement ( ) No lymphadenopathy **CV** ( ) PMI nondisplaced ( ) No murmur/ gallop/rub ( ) nl intensity w/o bruit ( ) No JVD ( ) nl femoral/pedal pulses ( ) No pedal edema	**Pulm** ( ) No retractions ( ) No dullness ( ) No fremitus ( ) No wheezing/ rales/rhonchi **GI** ( ) No masses/ tenderness ( ) No hep/ splenomegaly ( ) nl bowel sounds ( ) No dullness ( ) Heme (-) stool **GU** ( ) nl ext genitalia ( ) No hernia	**Neuro** ( ) AAO x 3 ( ) CN II-XII intact ( ) nl sensation ( ) Reflexes 2+ & symmetrical ( ) nl memory ( ) nl speech **MSK** ( ) nl tone ( ) nl bulk ( ) nl gait ( ) nl ROM UE ( ) nl ROM LE L___/5 UE R___/5 L___/5 LE R___/5

+ PE Findings

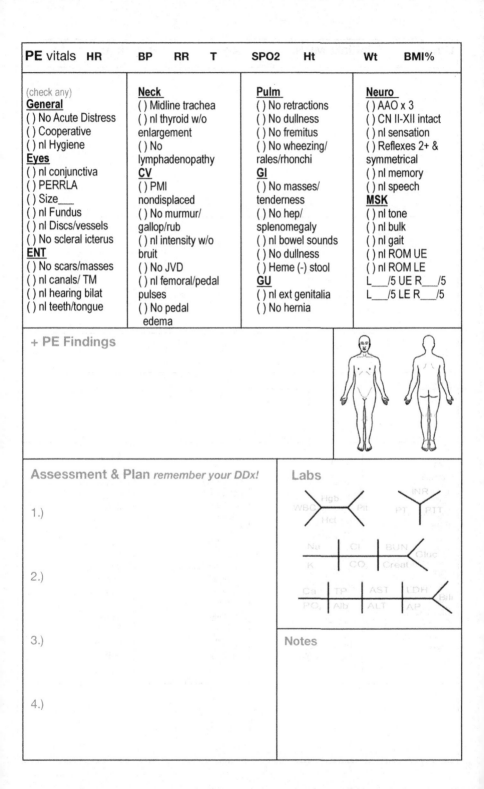

Assessment & Plan *remember your DDx!*

1.)

2.)

3.)

4.)

Labs

Notes

Date:	Initials/MRN:	Age:	Rotation:

CC: _____ y/o M/F
HPI: *symptoms/pertinent +/- ROS/prior episodes/recent travel/sick contacts*

PMHx *child/adult illness /hospitalizations/ immunizations*	**SurgHx** *type/when/ why/complications*	**FamHx** *parents/siblings/ children*

SHx *smoker/ETOH/illicits/exercise/sex/maritalstatus*

Allergies *meds/foods/ environmental/reactions*	**Meds** *reason/dose/time/route/compliance/vitamins/ herbs/otcs*

ROS (circle any)

Gen	**Pulm**	**GU**	**Endo**
Fatigue	Cough	Dysuria	Polyuria
Weight +/-	SOB	Frequency	Polydypsia
Chills	Wheezing	Hematuria	Polyphagia
Night sweats	Hemoptysis	Discharge	**Derm**
Eyes	**CV**	Flank pain	Rash
Pain	Chest pain	**MS**	Pruritis
Redness	Edema	Arthralgia	Wound(s)
Vision changes	PND	Arthritis	**Neuro**
ENT	Orthopnea	Joint swelling	Weakness
Headache	Palpitations	Myalgias	Seizures
Hoarseness	Claudication	Back pain	Parasthesias
Sore throat	**GI**	**Heme**	Tremors
Sinus sx	Abd pain	Bleeding	Syncope
Hearing loss	N/V	Bruising	**Psych**
Tinnitus	Heartburn	**Lymph**	Anxiety
Runny nose	Bloody stools	Swelling	Depression

+ ROS Findings

PE vitals	**HR**	**BP**	**RR**	**T**	**SPO2**	**Ht**	**Wt**	**BMI%**

(check any)

General
( ) No Acute Distress
( ) Cooperative
( ) nl Hygiene
Eyes
( ) nl conjunctiva
( ) PERRLA
( ) Size___
( ) nl Fundus
( ) nl Discs/vessels
( ) No scleral icterus
ENT
( ) No scars/masses
( ) nl canals/ TM
( ) nl hearing bilat
( ) nl teeth/tongue

Neck
( ) Midline trachea
( ) nl thyroid w/o enlargement
( ) No lymphadenopathy
CV
( ) PMI nondisplaced
( ) No murmur/ gallop/rub
( ) nl intensity w/o bruit
( ) No JVD
( ) nl femoral/pedal pulses
( ) No pedal edema

Pulm
( ) No retractions
( ) No dullness
( ) No fremitus
( ) No wheezing/ rales/rhonchi
GI
( ) No masses/ tenderness
( ) No hep/ splenomegaly
( ) nl bowel sounds
( ) No dullness
( ) Heme (-) stool
GU
( ) nl ext genitalia
( ) No hernia

Neuro
( ) AAO x 3
( ) CN II-XII intact
( ) nl sensation
( ) Reflexes 2+ & symmetrical
( ) nl memory
( ) nl speech
MSK
( ) nl tone
( ) nl bulk
( ) nl gait
( ) nl ROM UE
( ) nl ROM LE
L___/5 UE R___/5
L___/5 LE R___/5

+ PE Findings

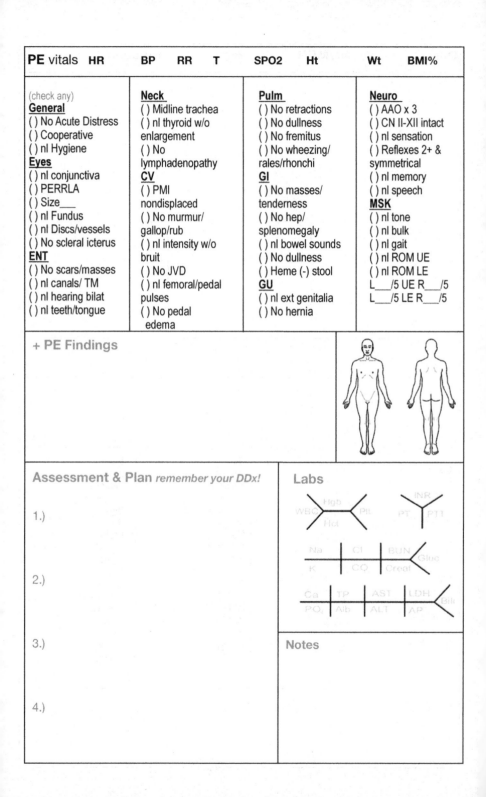

Assessment & Plan *remember your DDx!*

1.)

2.)

3.)

4.)

Labs

Notes

Date:	Initials/MRN:	Age:	Rotation:

CC: _____ y/o M/F
HPI: *symptoms/pertinent +/- ROS/prior episodes/recent travel/sick contacts*

PMHx *child/adult illness /hospitalizations/ immunizations*

SurgHx *type/when/ why/complications*

FamHx *parents/siblings/ children*

SHx *smoker/ETOH/illicits/exercise/sex/maritalstatus*

Allergies *meds/foods/ environmental/reactions*

Meds *reason/dose/time/route/compliance/vitamins/ herbs/otcs*

ROS (circle any)

Gen
Fatigue
Weight +/-
Chills
Night sweats
Eyes
Pain
Redness
Vision changes
ENT
Headache
Hoarseness
Sore throat
Sinus sx
Hearing loss
Tinnitus
Runny nose

Pulm
Cough
SOB
Wheezing
Hemoptysis
CV
Chest pain
Edema
PND
Orthopnea
Palpitations
Claudication
GI
Abd pain
N/V
Heartburn
Bloody stools

GU
Dysuria
Frequency
Hematuria
Discharge
Flank pain
MS
Arthralgia
Arthritis
Joint swelling
Myalgias
Back pain
Heme
Bleeding
Bruising
Lymph
Swelling

Endo
Polyuria
Polydypsia
Polyphagia
Derm
Rash
Pruritis
Wound(s)
Neuro
Weakness
Seizures
Parasthesias
Tremors
Syncope
Psych
Anxiety
Depression

+ ROS Findings

PE vitals **HR**   **BP**   **RR**   **T**   **SPO2**   **Ht**   **Wt**   **BMI%**

(check any) **General** ( ) No Acute Distress ( ) Cooperative ( ) nl Hygiene **Eyes** ( ) nl conjunctiva ( ) PERRLA ( ) Size___ ( ) nl Fundus ( ) nl Discs/vessels ( ) No scleral icterus **ENT** ( ) No scars/masses ( ) nl canals/ TM ( ) nl hearing bilat ( ) nl teeth/tongue	**Neck** ( ) Midline trachea ( ) nl thyroid w/o enlargement ( ) No lymphadenopathy **CV** ( ) PMI nondisplaced ( ) No murmur/ gallop/rub ( ) nl intensity w/o bruit ( ) No JVD ( ) nl femoral/pedal pulses ( ) No pedal edema	**Pulm** ( ) No retractions ( ) No dullness ( ) No fremitus ( ) No wheezing/ rales/rhonchi **GI** ( ) No masses/ tenderness ( ) No hep/ splenomegaly ( ) nl bowel sounds ( ) No dullness ( ) Heme (-) stool **GU** ( ) nl ext genitalia ( ) No hernia	**Neuro** ( ) AAO x 3 ( ) CN II-XII intact ( ) nl sensation ( ) Reflexes 2+ & symmetrical ( ) nl memory ( ) nl speech **MSK** ( ) nl tone ( ) nl bulk ( ) nl gait ( ) nl ROM UE ( ) nl ROM LE L___/5 UE R___/5 L___/5 LE R___/5

+ PE Findings

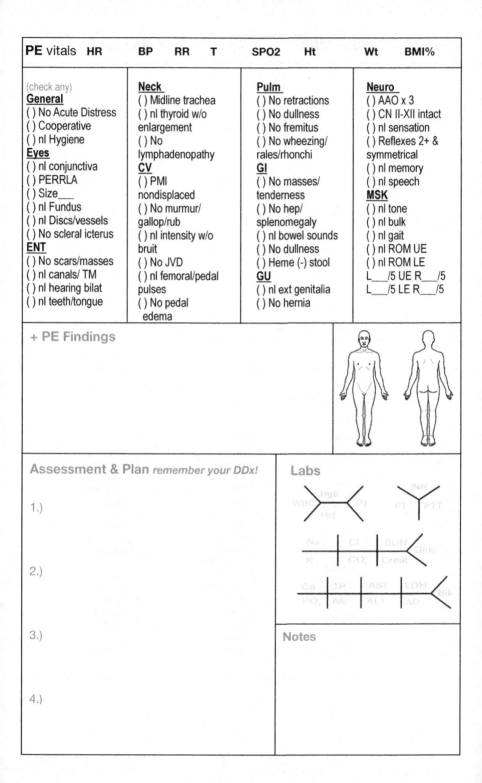

Assessment & Plan *remember your DDx!*

1.)

2.)

3.)

4.)

Labs

Hgb
WBC   Plt
Hct

INR
PT   PTT

Na | Cl | BUN
K | CO₂ | Creat Gluc

Ca | TP | AST | LDH
PO₄ | Alb | ALT | AP Bili

Notes

Date: **Initials/MRN:**   **Age:**   **Rotation:**

CC: _____ y/o M/F
HPI: *symptoms/pertinent +/- ROS/prior episodes/recent travel/sick contacts*

PMHx *child/adult illness /hospitalizations/ immunizations*

SurgHx *type/when/ why/complications*

FamHx *parents/siblings/ children*

SHx *smoker/ETOH/illicits/exercise/sex/maritalstatus*

Allergies *meds/foods/ environmental/reactions*

Meds *reason/dose/time/route/compliance/vitamins/ herbs/otcs*

ROS (circle any)

Gen	**Pulm**	**GU**	**Endo**
Fatigue	Cough	Dysuria	Polyuria
Weight +/-	SOB	Frequency	Polydypsia
Chills	Wheezing	Hematuria	Polyphagia
Night sweats	Hemoptysis	Discharge	**Derm**
Eyes	**CV**	Flank pain	Rash
Pain	Chest pain	**MS**	Pruritis
Redness	Edema	Arthralgia	Wound(s)
Vision changes	PND	Arthritis	**Neuro**
ENT	Orthopnea	Joint swelling	Weakness
Headache	Palpitations	Myalgias	Seizures
Hoarseness	Claudication	Back pain	Parasthesias
Sore throat	**GI**	**Heme**	Tremors
Sinus sx	Abd pain	Bleeding	Syncope
Hearing loss	N/V	Bruising	**Psych**
Tinnitus	Heartburn	**Lymph**	Anxiety
Runny nose	Bloody stools	Swelling	Depression

+ ROS Findings

PE vitals   HR   BP   RR   T   SPO2   Ht   Wt   BMI%

General (check any)	Neck	Pulm	Neuro
( ) No Acute Distress	( ) Midline trachea	( ) No retractions	( ) AAO x 3
( ) Cooperative	( ) nl thyroid w/o	( ) No dullness	( ) CN II-XII intact
( ) nl Hygiene	enlargement	( ) No fremitus	( ) nl sensation
Eyes	( ) No	( ) No wheezing/	( ) Reflexes 2+ &
( ) nl conjunctiva	lymphadenopathy	rales/rhonchi	symmetrical
( ) PERRLA	**CV**	**GI**	( ) nl memory
( ) Size___	( ) PMI	( ) No masses/	( ) nl speech
( ) nl Fundus	nondisplaced	tenderness	**MSK**
( ) nl Discs/vessels	( ) No murmur/	( ) No hep/	( ) nl tone
( ) No scleral icterus	gallop/rub	splenomegaly	( ) nl bulk
ENT	( ) nl intensity w/o	( ) nl bowel sounds	( ) nl gait
( ) No scars/masses	bruit	( ) No dullness	( ) nl ROM UE
( ) nl canals/ TM	( ) No JVD	( ) Heme (-) stool	( ) nl ROM LE
( ) nl hearing bilat	( ) nl femoral/pedal	**GU**	L___/5 UE R___/5
( ) nl teeth/tongue	pulses	( ) nl ext genitalia	L___/5 LE R___/5
	( ) No pedal	( ) No hernia	
	edema		

+ PE Findings

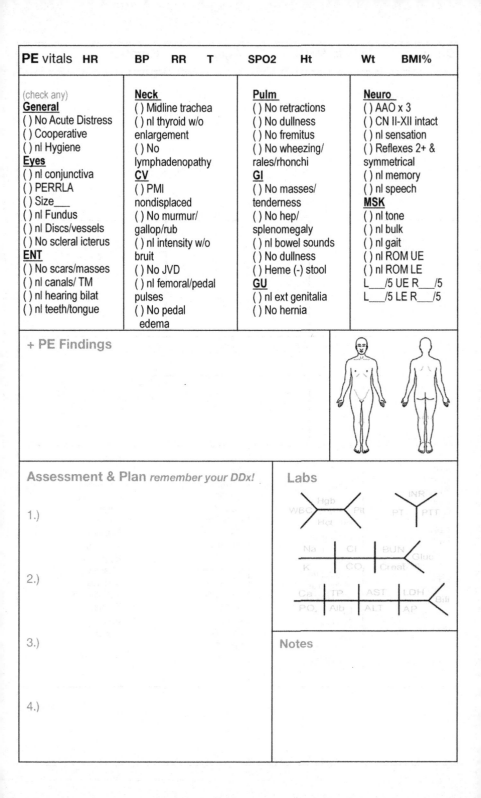

Assessment & Plan *remember your DDx!*

1.)

2.)

3.)

4.)

Labs

Notes

Date:	Initials/MRN:	Age:	Rotation:

CC: _____ y/o M/F
HPI: *symptoms/pertinent +/- ROS/prior episodes/recent travel/sick contacts*

PMHx *child/adult illness /hospitalizations/ immunizations*	**SurgHx** *type/when/ why/complications*	**FamHx** *parents/siblings/ children*

SHx *smoker/ETOH/illicits/exercise/sex/maritalstatus*

Allergies *meds/foods/ environmental/reactions*	**Meds** *reason/dose/time/route/compliance/vitamins/ herbs/otcs*

ROS (circle any)

Gen	**Pulm**	**GU**	**Endo**
Fatigue	Cough	Dysuria	Polyuria
Weight +/-	SOB	Frequency	Polydypsia
Chills	Wheezing	Hematuria	Polyphagia
Night sweats	Hemoptysis	Discharge	**Derm**
Eyes	**CV**	Flank pain	Rash
Pain	Chest pain	**MS**	Pruritis
Redness	Edema	Arthralgia	Wound(s)
Vision changes	PND	Arthritis	**Neuro**
ENT	Orthopnea	Joint swelling	Weakness
Headache	Palpitations	Myalgias	Seizures
Hoarseness	Claudication	Back pain	Parasthesias
Sore throat	**GI**	**Heme**	Tremors
Sinus sx	Abd pain	Bleeding	Syncope
Hearing loss	N/V	Bruising	**Psych**
Tinnitus	Heartburn	**Lymph**	Anxiety
Runny nose	Bloody stools	Swelling	Depression

+ ROS Findings

PE vitals	HR	BP	RR	T	SPO2	Ht	Wt	BMI%

(check any)	**Neck**	**Pulm**	**Neuro**
General	( ) Midline trachea	( ) No retractions	( ) AAO x 3
( ) No Acute Distress	( ) nl thyroid w/o	( ) No dullness	( ) CN II-XII intact
( ) Cooperative	enlargement	( ) No fremitus	( ) nl sensation
( ) nl Hygiene	( ) No	( ) No wheezing/	( ) Reflexes 2+ &
Eyes	lymphadenopathy	rales/rhonchi	symmetrical
( ) nl conjunctiva	**CV**	**GI**	( ) nl memory
( ) PERRLA	( ) PMI	( ) No masses/	( ) nl speech
( ) Size___	nondisplaced	tenderness	**MSK**
( ) nl Fundus	( ) No murmur/	( ) No hep/	( ) nl tone
( ) nl Discs/vessels	gallop/rub	splenomegaly	( ) nl bulk
( ) No scleral icterus	( ) nl intensity w/o	( ) nl bowel sounds	( ) nl gait
ENT	bruit	( ) No dullness	( ) nl ROM UE
( ) No scars/masses	( ) No JVD	( ) Heme (-) stool	( ) nl ROM LE
( ) nl canals/ TM	( ) nl femoral/pedal	**GU**	L___/5 UE R___/5
( ) nl hearing bilat	pulses	( ) nl ext genitalia	L___/5 LE R___/5
( ) nl teeth/tongue	( ) No pedal	( ) No hernia	
	edema		

+ PE Findings

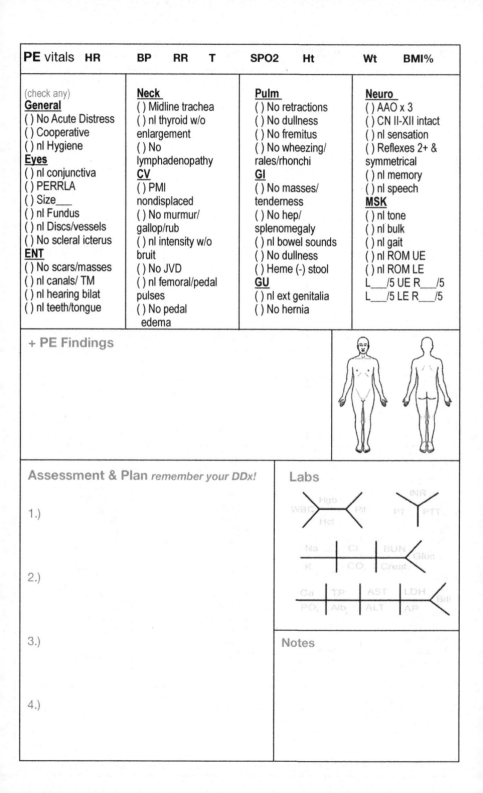

Assessment & Plan *remember your DDx!*

1.)

2.)

3.)

4.)

Labs

Notes

Date:	Initials/MRN:	Age:	Rotation:

CC: _____ y/o M/F
HPI: *symptoms/pertinent +/- ROS/prior episodes/recent travel/sick contacts*

PMHx *child/adult illness /hospitalizations/ immunizations*

SurgHx *type/when/ why/complications*

FamHx *parents/siblings/ children*

SHx *smoker/ETOH/illicits/exercise/sex/maritalstatus*

Allergies *meds/foods/ environmental/reactions*

Meds *reason/dose/time/route/compliance/vitamins/ herbs/otcs*

ROS (circle any)

Gen	**Pulm**	**GU**	**Endo**
Fatigue	Cough	Dysuria	Polyuria
Weight +/-	SOB	Frequency	Polydypsia
Chills	Wheezing	Hematuria	Polyphagia
Night sweats	Hemoptysis	Discharge	**Derm**
Eyes	**CV**	Flank pain	Rash
Pain	Chest pain	**MS**	Pruritis
Redness	Edema	Arthralgia	Wound(s)
Vision changes	PND	Arthritis	**Neuro**
ENT	Orthopnea	Joint swelling	Weakness
Headache	Palpitations	Myalgias	Seizures
Hoarseness	Claudication	Back pain	Parasthesias
Sore throat	**GI**	**Heme**	Tremors
Sinus sx	Abd pain	Bleeding	Syncope
Hearing loss	N/V	Bruising	**Psych**
Tinnitus	Heartburn	**Lymph**	Anxiety
Runny nose	Bloody stools	Swelling	Depression

+ ROS Findings

PE vitals	HR	BP	RR	T	SPO2	Ht	Wt	BMI%

(check any)

General
( ) No Acute Distress
( ) Cooperative
( ) nl Hygiene

Eyes
( ) nl conjunctiva
( ) PERRLA
( ) Size___
( ) nl Fundus
( ) nl Discs/vessels
( ) No scleral icterus

ENT
( ) No scars/masses
( ) nl canals/ TM
( ) nl hearing bilat
( ) nl teeth/tongue

Neck
( ) Midline trachea
( ) nl thyroid w/o enlargement
( ) No lymphadenopathy

CV
( ) PMI nondisplaced
( ) No murmur/ gallop/rub
( ) nl intensity w/o bruit
( ) No JVD
( ) nl femoral/pedal pulses
( ) No pedal edema

Pulm
( ) No retractions
( ) No dullness
( ) No fremitus
( ) No wheezing/ rales/rhonchi

GI
( ) No masses/ tenderness
( ) No hep/ splenomegaly
( ) nl bowel sounds
( ) No dullness
( ) Heme (-) stool

GU
( ) nl ext genitalia
( ) No hernia

Neuro
( ) AAO x 3
( ) CN II-XII intact
( ) nl sensation
( ) Reflexes 2+ & symmetrical
( ) nl memory
( ) nl speech

MSK
( ) nl tone
( ) nl bulk
( ) nl gait
( ) nl ROM UE
( ) nl ROM LE
L___/5 UE R___/5
L___/5 LE R___/5

+ PE Findings

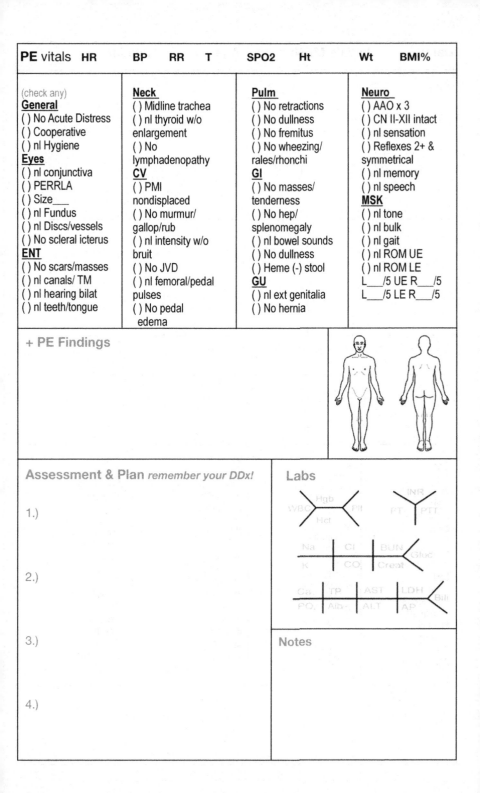

Assessment & Plan *remember your DDx!*

1.)

2.)

3.)

4.)

Labs

Hgb
WBC   Plt
       Hct

Na   Cl   BUN
               Gluc
K   CO₂   Creat

INR
PT   PTT

Ca   TP   AST   LDH
                        Bili
PO₄   Alb-   ALT   AP

Notes

Date:	Initials/MRN:	Age:	Rotation:

CC: _____ y/o M/F
HPI: *symptoms/pertinent +/- ROS/prior episodes/recent travel/sick contacts*

PMHx *child/adult illness /hospitalizations/ immunizations*

SurgHx *type/when/ why/complications*

FamHx *parents/siblings/ children*

SHx *smoker/ETOH/illicits/exercise/sex/maritalstatus*

Allergies *meds/foods/ environmental/reactions*

Meds *reason/dose/time/route/compliance/vitamins/ herbs/otcs*

ROS (circle any)

Gen	**Pulm**	**GU**	**Endo**
Fatigue	Cough	Dysuria	Polyuria
Weight +/-	SOB	Frequency	Polydypsia
Chills	Wheezing	Hematuria	Polyphagia
Night sweats	Hemoptysis	Discharge	**Derm**
Eyes	**CV**	Flank pain	Rash
Pain	Chest pain	**MS**	Pruritis
Redness	Edema	Arthralgia	Wound(s)
Vision changes	PND	Arthritis	**Neuro**
ENT	Orthopnea	Joint swelling	Weakness
Headache	Palpitations	Myalgias	Seizures
Hoarseness	Claudication	Back pain	Parasthesias
Sore throat	**GI**	**Heme**	Tremors
Sinus sx	Abd pain	Bleeding	Syncope
Hearing loss	N/V	Bruising	**Psych**
Tinnitus	Heartburn	**Lymph**	Anxiety
Runny nose	Bloody stools	Swelling	Depression

+ ROS Findings

PE vitals   HR   BP   RR   T   SPO2   Ht   Wt   BMI%

(check any)	**Neck**	**Pulm**	**Neuro**
General	( ) Midline trachea	( ) No retractions	( ) AAO x 3
( ) No Acute Distress	( ) nl thyroid w/o	( ) No dullness	( ) CN II-XII intact
( ) Cooperative	enlargement	( ) No fremitus	( ) nl sensation
( ) nl Hygiene	( ) No	( ) No wheezing/	( ) Reflexes 2+ &
Eyes	lymphadenopathy	rales/rhonchi	symmetrical
( ) nl conjunctiva	**CV**	**GI**	( ) nl memory
( ) PERRLA	( ) PMI	( ) No masses/	( ) nl speech
( ) Size___	nondisplaced	tenderness	**MSK**
( ) nl Fundus	( ) No murmur/	( ) No hep/	( ) nl tone
( ) nl Discs/vessels	gallop/rub	splenomegaly	( ) nl bulk
( ) No scleral icterus	( ) nl intensity w/o	( ) nl bowel sounds	( ) nl gait
ENT	bruit	( ) No dullness	( ) nl ROM UE
( ) No scars/masses	( ) No JVD	( ) Heme (-) stool	( ) nl ROM LE
( ) nl canals/ TM	( ) nl femoral/pedal	**GU**	L___/5 UE R___/5
( ) nl hearing bilat	pulses	( ) nl ext genitalia	L___/5 LE R___/5
( ) nl teeth/tongue	( ) No pedal	( ) No hernia	
	edema		

+ PE Findings

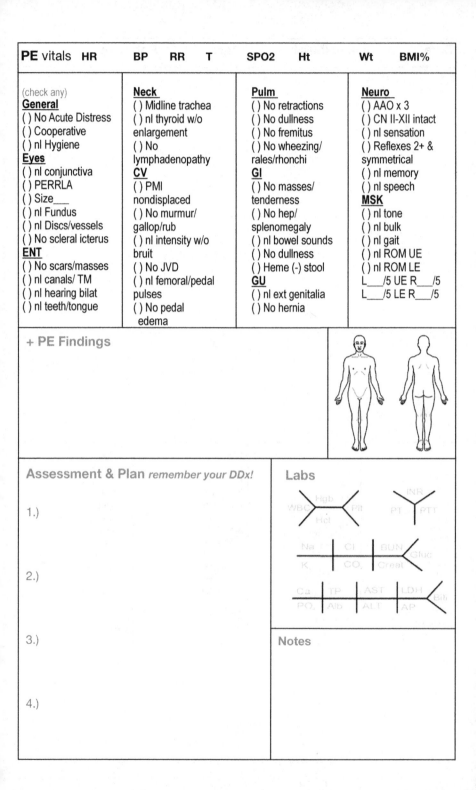

Assessment & Plan *remember your DDx!*

1.)

2.)

3.)

4.)

Labs

Notes

Date:	Initials/MRN:	Age:	Rotation:

CC: _____ y/o M/F
HPI: *symptoms/pertinent +/- ROS/prior episodes/recent travel/sick contacts*

PMHx *child/adult illness /hospitalizations/ immunizations*	**SurgHx** *type/when/ why/complications*	**FamHx** *parents/siblings/ children*

SHx *smoker/ETOH/illicits/exercise/sex/maritalstatus*

Allergies *meds/foods/ environmental/reactions*	**Meds** *reason/dose/time/route/compliance/vitamins/ herbs/otcs*

ROS (circle any)

Gen Fatigue Weight +/- Chills Night sweats **Eyes** Pain Redness Vision changes **ENT** Headache Hoarseness Sore throat Sinus sx Hearing loss Tinnitus Runny nose	**Pulm** Cough SOB Wheezing Hemoptysis **CV** Chest pain Edema PND Orthopnea Palpitations Claudication **GI** Abd pain N/V Heartburn Bloody stools	**GU** Dysuria Frequency Hematuria Discharge Flank pain **MS** Arthralgia Arthritis Joint swelling Myalgias Back pain **Heme** Bleeding Bruising **Lymph** Swelling	**Endo** Polyuria Polydypsia Polyphagia **Derm** Rash Pruritis Wound(s) **Neuro** Weakness Seizures Parasthesias Tremors Syncope **Psych** Anxiety Depression

+ ROS Findings

PE vitals	HR	BP	RR	T	SPO2	Ht	Wt	BMI%

(check any)

General
( ) No Acute Distress
( ) Cooperative
( ) nl Hygiene
Eyes
( ) nl conjunctiva
( ) PERRLA
( ) Size___
( ) nl Fundus
( ) nl Discs/vessels
( ) No scleral icterus
ENT
( ) No scars/masses
( ) nl canals/ TM
( ) nl hearing bilat
( ) nl teeth/tongue

Neck
( ) Midline trachea
( ) nl thyroid w/o
enlargement
( ) No
lymphadenopathy
CV
( ) PMI
nondisplaced
( ) No murmur/
gallop/rub
( ) nl intensity w/o
bruit
( ) No JVD
( ) nl femoral/pedal
pulses
( ) No pedal
  edema

Pulm
( ) No retractions
( ) No dullness
( ) No fremitus
( ) No wheezing/
rales/rhonchi
GI
( ) No masses/
tenderness
( ) No hep/
splenomegaly
( ) nl bowel sounds
( ) No dullness
( ) Heme (-) stool
GU
( ) nl ext genitalia
( ) No hernia

Neuro
( ) AAO x 3
( ) CN II-XII intact
( ) nl sensation
( ) Reflexes 2+ &
symmetrical
( ) nl memory
( ) nl speech
MSK
( ) nl tone
( ) nl bulk
( ) nl gait
( ) nl ROM UE
( ) nl ROM LE
L___/5 UE R___/5
L___/5 LE R___/5

+ PE Findings

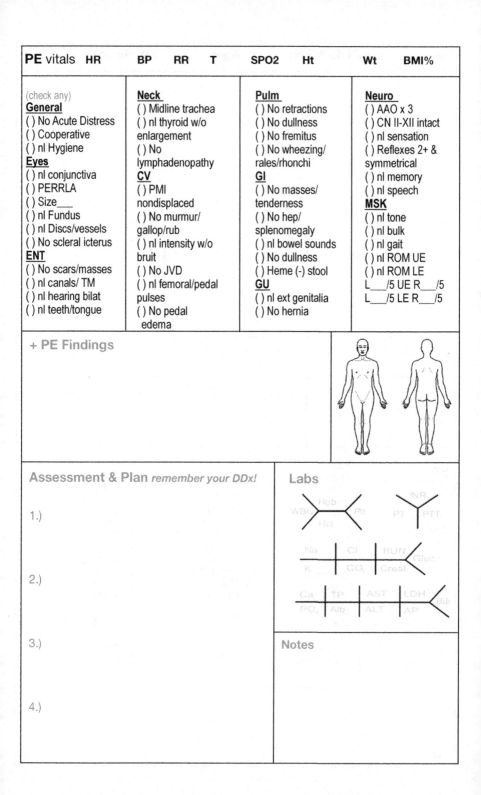

Assessment & Plan *remember your DDx!*

1.)

2.)

3.)

4.)

Labs

Notes

Date:	Initials/MRN:	Age:	Rotation:

CC: _____ y/o M/F
HPI: *symptoms/pertinent +/- ROS/prior episodes/recent travel/sick contacts*

PMHx *child/adult illness /hospitalizations/ immunizations*

SurgHx *type/when/ why/complications*

FamHx *parents/siblings/ children*

SHx *smoker/ETOH/illicits/exercise/sex/maritalstatus*

Allergies *meds/foods/ environmental/reactions*

Meds *reason/dose/time/route/compliance/vitamins/ herbs/otcs*

ROS (circle any)

Gen	**Pulm**	**GU**	**Endo**
Fatigue	Cough	Dysuria	Polyuria
Weight +/-	SOB	Frequency	Polydypsia
Chills	Wheezing	Hematuria	Polyphagia
Night sweats	Hemoptysis	Discharge	**Derm**
Eyes	**CV**	Flank pain	Rash
Pain	Chest pain	**MS**	Pruritis
Redness	Edema	Arthralgia	Wound(s)
Vision changes	PND	Arthritis	**Neuro**
ENT	Orthopnea	Joint swelling	Weakness
Headache	Palpitations	Myalgias	Seizures
Hoarseness	Claudication	Back pain	Parasthesias
Sore throat	**GI**	**Heme**	Tremors
Sinus sx	Abd pain	Bleeding	Syncope
Hearing loss	N/V	Bruising	**Psych**
Tinnitus	Heartburn	**Lymph**	Anxiety
Runny nose	Bloody stools	Swelling	Depression

+ ROS Findings

PE vitals	HR	BP	RR	T	SPO2	Ht	Wt	BMI%

(check any)	**Neck**	**Pulm**	**Neuro**
General	( ) Midline trachea	( ) No retractions	( ) AAO x 3
( ) No Acute Distress	( ) nl thyroid w/o	( ) No dullness	( ) CN II-XII intact
( ) Cooperative	enlargement	( ) No fremitus	( ) nl sensation
( ) nl Hygiene	( ) No	( ) No wheezing/	( ) Reflexes 2+ &
Eyes	lymphadenopathy	rales/rhonchi	symmetrical
( ) nl conjunctiva	**CV**	**GI**	( ) nl memory
( ) PERRLA	( ) PMI	( ) No masses/	( ) nl speech
( ) Size___	nondisplaced	tenderness	**MSK**
( ) nl Fundus	( ) No murmur/	( ) No hep/	( ) nl tone
( ) nl Discs/vessels	gallop/rub	splenomegaly	( ) nl bulk
( ) No scleral icterus	( ) nl intensity w/o	( ) nl bowel sounds	( ) nl gait
ENT	bruit	( ) No dullness	( ) nl ROM UE
( ) No scars/masses	( ) No JVD	( ) Heme (-) stool	( ) nl ROM LE
( ) nl canals/ TM	( ) nl femoral/pedal	**GU**	L___/5 UE R___/5
( ) nl hearing bilat	pulses	( ) nl ext genitalia	L___/5 LE R___/5
( ) nl teeth/tongue	( ) No pedal	( ) No hernia	
	edema		

+ PE Findings

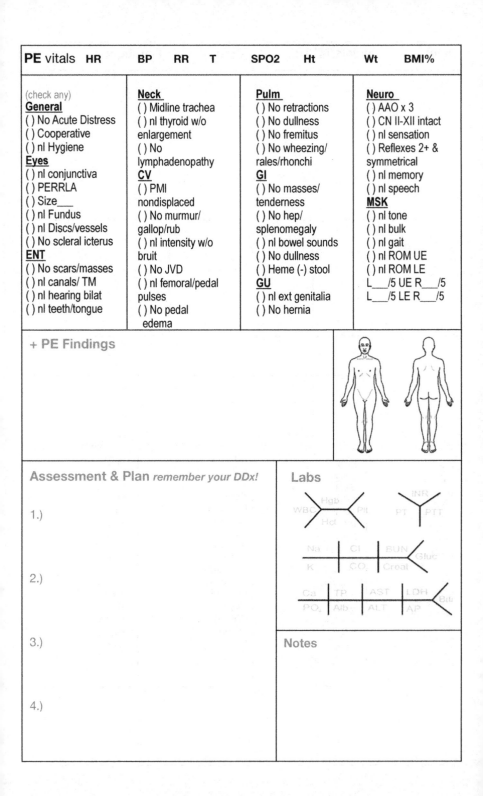

Assessment & Plan *remember your DDx!*

1.)

2.)

3.)

4.)

Labs

Notes

Date:	Initials/MRN:	Age:	Rotation:

CC: _____ y/o M/F
HPI: *symptoms/pertinent +/- ROS/prior episodes/recent travel/sick contacts*

PMHx *child/adult illness /hospitalizations/ immunizations*	**SurgHx** *type/when/ why/complications*	**FamHx** *parents/siblings/ children*

SHx *smoker/ETOH/illicits/exercise/sex/maritalstatus*

Allergies *meds/foods/ environmental/reactions*	**Meds** *reason/dose/time/route/compliance/vitamins/ herbs/otcs*

ROS (circle any)

Gen	**Pulm**	**GU**	**Endo**
Fatigue	Cough	Dysuria	Polyuria
Weight +/-	SOB	Frequency	Polydypsia
Chills	Wheezing	Hematuria	Polyphagia
Night sweats	Hemoptysis	Discharge	**Derm**
Eyes	**CV**	Flank pain	Rash
Pain	Chest pain	**MS**	Pruritis
Redness	Edema	Arthralgia	Wound(s)
Vision changes	PND	Arthritis	**Neuro**
ENT	Orthopnea	Joint swelling	Weakness
Headache	Palpitations	Myalgias	Seizures
Hoarseness	Claudication	Back pain	Parasthesias
Sore throat	**GI**	**Heme**	Tremors
Sinus sx	Abd pain	Bleeding	Syncope
Hearing loss	N/V	Bruising	**Psych**
Tinnitus	Heartburn	**Lymph**	Anxiety
Runny nose	Bloody stools	Swelling	Depression

+ ROS Findings

PE vitals HR   BP   RR   T   SPO2   Ht   Wt   BMI%

(check any)	**Neck**	**Pulm**	**Neuro**
General	( ) Midline trachea	( ) No retractions	( ) AAO x 3
( ) No Acute Distress	( ) nl thyroid w/o	( ) No dullness	( ) CN II-XII intact
( ) Cooperative	enlargement	( ) No fremitus	( ) nl sensation
( ) nl Hygiene	( ) No	( ) No wheezing/	( ) Reflexes 2+ &
Eyes	lymphadenopathy	rales/rhonchi	symmetrical
( ) nl conjunctiva	**CV**	**GI**	( ) nl memory
( ) PERRLA	( ) PMI	( ) No masses/	( ) nl speech
( ) Size___	nondisplaced	tenderness	**MSK**
( ) nl Fundus	( ) No murmur/	( ) No hep/	( ) nl tone
( ) nl Discs/vessels	gallop/rub	splenomegaly	( ) nl bulk
( ) No scleral icterus	( ) nl intensity w/o	( ) nl bowel sounds	( ) nl gait
ENT	bruit	( ) No dullness	( ) nl ROM UE
( ) No scars/masses	( ) No JVD	( ) Heme (-) stool	( ) nl ROM LE
( ) nl canals/ TM	( ) nl femoral/pedal	**GU**	L___/5 UE R___/5
( ) nl hearing bilat	pulses	( ) nl ext genitalia	L___/5 LE R___/5
( ) nl teeth/tongue	( ) No pedal	( ) No hernia	
	edema		

+ PE Findings

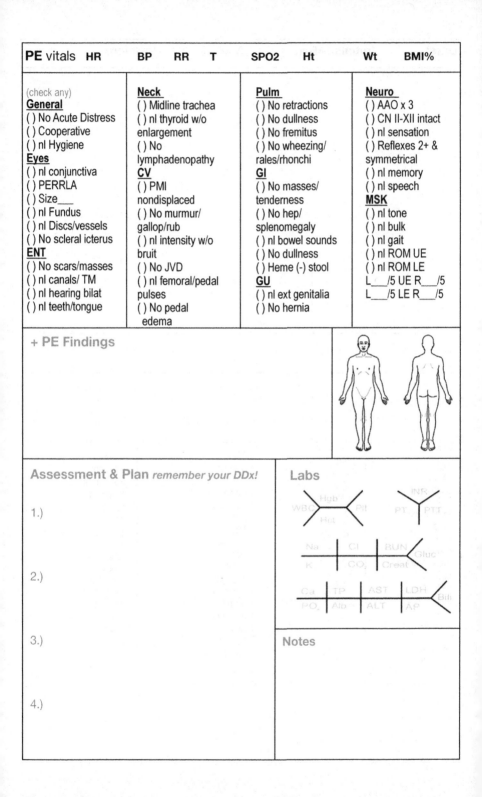

Assessment & Plan *remember your DDx!*

1.)

2.)

3.)

4.)

Labs

Notes

Date:	Initials/MRN:	Age:	Rotation:

CC: _____ y/o M/F
HPI: *symptoms/pertinent +/- ROS/prior episodes/recent travel/sick contacts*

PMHx *child/adult illness /hospitalizations/ immunizations*

SurgHx *type/when/ why/complications*

FamHx *parents/siblings/ children*

SHx *smoker/ETOH/illicits/exercise/sex/maritalstatus*

Allergies *meds/foods/ environmental/reactions*

Meds *reason/dose/time/route/compliance/vitamins/ herbs/otcs*

ROS (circle any)

Gen
Fatigue
Weight +/-
Chills
Night sweats
Eyes
Pain
Redness
Vision changes
ENT
Headache
Hoarseness
Sore throat
Sinus sx
Hearing loss
Tinnitus
Runny nose

Pulm
Cough
SOB
Wheezing
Hemoptysis
CV
Chest pain
Edema
PND
Orthopnea
Palpitations
Claudication
GI
Abd pain
N/V
Heartburn
Bloody stools

GU
Dysuria
Frequency
Hematuria
Discharge
Flank pain
MS
Arthralgia
Arthritis
Joint swelling
Myalgias
Back pain
Heme
Bleeding
Bruising
Lymph
Swelling

Endo
Polyuria
Polydypsia
Polyphagia
Derm
Rash
Pruritis
Wound(s)
Neuro
Weakness
Seizures
Parasthesias
Tremors
Syncope
Psych
Anxiety
Depression

+ ROS Findings

PE vitals   **HR**   **BP**   **RR**   **T**   **SPO2**   **Ht**   **Wt**   **BMI%**

(check any)	**Neck**	**Pulm**	**Neuro**
General	( ) Midline trachea	( ) No retractions	( ) AAO x 3
( ) No Acute Distress	( ) nl thyroid w/o	( ) No dullness	( ) CN II-XII intact
( ) Cooperative	enlargement	( ) No fremitus	( ) nl sensation
( ) nl Hygiene	( ) No	( ) No wheezing/	( ) Reflexes 2+ &
Eyes	lymphadenopathy	rales/rhonchi	symmetrical
( ) nl conjunctiva	**CV**	**GI**	( ) nl memory
( ) PERRLA	( ) PMI	( ) No masses/	( ) nl speech
( ) Size___	nondisplaced	tenderness	**MSK**
( ) nl Fundus	( ) No murmur/	( ) No hep/	( ) nl tone
( ) nl Discs/vessels	gallop/rub	splenomegaly	( ) nl bulk
( ) No scleral icterus	( ) nl intensity w/o	( ) nl bowel sounds	( ) nl gait
ENT	bruit	( ) No dullness	( ) nl ROM UE
( ) No scars/masses	( ) No JVD	( ) Heme (-) stool	( ) nl ROM LE
( ) nl canals/ TM	( ) nl femoral/pedal	**GU**	L___/5 UE R___/5
( ) nl hearing bilat	pulses	( ) nl ext genitalia	L___/5 LE R___/5
( ) nl teeth/tongue	( ) No pedal	( ) No hernia	
	edema		

+ PE Findings

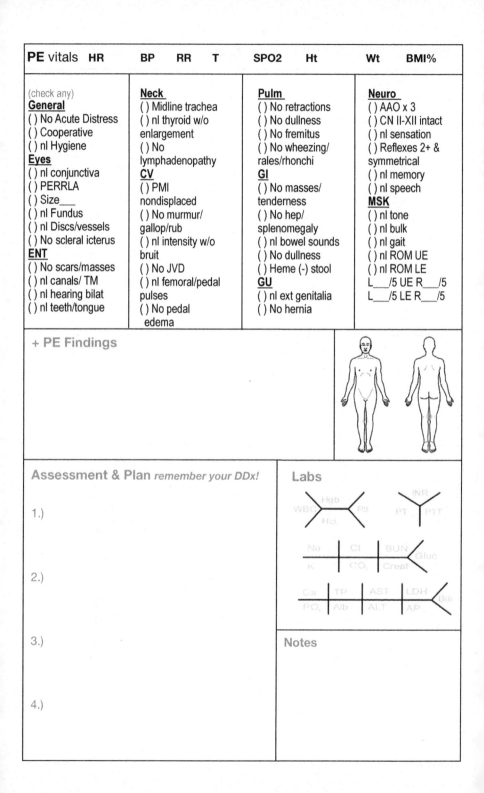

Assessment & Plan *remember your DDx!*

1.)

2.)

3.)

4.)

Labs

Notes

Date:	Initials/MRN:	Age:	Rotation:

CC: _____ y/o M/F
HPI: *symptoms/pertinent +/- ROS/prior episodes/recent travel/sick contacts*

PMHx *child/adult illness /hospitalizations/ immunizations*	**SurgHx** *type/when/ why/complications*	**FamHx** *parents/siblings/ children*

SHx *smoker/ETOH/illicits/exercise/sex/maritalstatus*

Allergies *meds/foods/ environmental/reactions*	**Meds** *reason/dose/time/route/compliance/vitamins/ herbs/otcs*

ROS (circle any)

Gen	**Pulm**	**GU**	**Endo**
Fatigue	Cough	Dysuria	Polyuria
Weight +/-	SOB	Frequency	Polydypsia
Chills	Wheezing	Hematuria	Polyphagia
Night sweats	Hemoptysis	Discharge	**Derm**
Eyes	**CV**	Flank pain	Rash
Pain	Chest pain	**MS**	Pruritis
Redness	Edema	Arthralgia	Wound(s)
Vision changes	PND	Arthritis	**Neuro**
ENT	Orthopnea	Joint swelling	Weakness
Headache	Palpitations	Myalgias	Seizures
Hoarseness	Claudication	Back pain	Parasthesias
Sore throat	**GI**	**Heme**	Tremors
Sinus sx	Abd pain	Bleeding	Syncope
Hearing loss	N/V	Bruising	**Psych**
Tinnitus	Heartburn	**Lymph**	Anxiety
Runny nose	Bloody stools	Swelling	Depression

+ ROS Findings

PE vitals **HR**	**BP** **RR** **T**	**SPO2** **Ht**	**Wt** **BMI%**

(check any)	**Neck**	**Pulm**	**Neuro**
General	( ) Midline trachea	( ) No retractions	( ) AAO x 3
( ) No Acute Distress	( ) nl thyroid w/o	( ) No dullness	( ) CN II-XII intact
( ) Cooperative	enlargement	( ) No fremitus	( ) nl sensation
( ) nl Hygiene	( ) No	( ) No wheezing/	( ) Reflexes 2+ &
Eyes	lymphadenopathy	rales/rhonchi	symmetrical
( ) nl conjunctiva	**CV**	**GI**	( ) nl memory
( ) PERRLA	( ) PMI	( ) No masses/	( ) nl speech
( ) Size___	nondisplaced	tenderness	**MSK**
( ) nl Fundus	( ) No murmur/	( ) No hep/	( ) nl tone
( ) nl Discs/vessels	gallop/rub	splenomegaly	( ) nl bulk
( ) No scleral icterus	( ) nl intensity w/o	( ) nl bowel sounds	( ) nl gait
ENT	bruit	( ) No dullness	( ) nl ROM UE
( ) No scars/masses	( ) No JVD	( ) Heme (-) stool	( ) nl ROM LE
( ) nl canals/ TM	( ) nl femoral/pedal	**GU**	L___/5 UE R___/5
( ) nl hearing bilat	pulses	( ) nl ext genitalia	L___/5 LE R___/5
( ) nl teeth/tongue	( ) No pedal	( ) No hernia	
	edema		

+ PE Findings

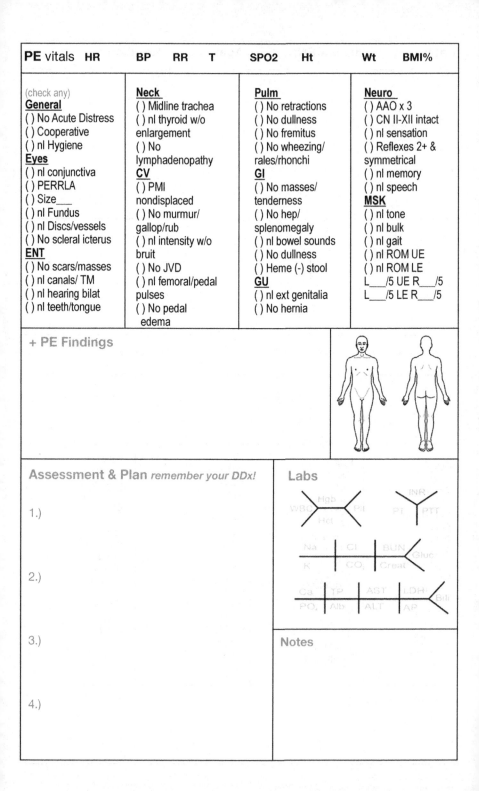

Assessment & Plan *remember your DDx!*

1.)

2.)

3.)

4.)

Labs

Notes

Date:	Initials/MRN:	Age:	Rotation:

CC: _____ y/o M/F
HPI: *symptoms/pertinent +/- ROS/prior episodes/recent travel/sick contacts*

PMHx *child/adult illness /hospitalizations/ immunizations*

SurgHx *type/when/ why/complications*

FamHx *parents/siblings/ children*

SHx *smoker/ETOH/illicits/exercise/sex/maritalstatus*

Allergies *meds/foods/ environmental/reactions*

Meds *reason/dose/time/route/compliance/vitamins/ herbs/otcs*

ROS (circle any)

Gen
Fatigue
Weight +/-
Chills
Night sweats
Eyes
Pain
Redness
Vision changes
ENT
Headache
Hoarseness
Sore throat
Sinus sx
Hearing loss
Tinnitus
Runny nose

Pulm
Cough
SOB
Wheezing
Hemoptysis
CV
Chest pain
Edema
PND
Orthopnea
Palpitations
Claudication
GI
Abd pain
N/V
Heartburn
Bloody stools

GU
Dysuria
Frequency
Hematuria
Discharge
Flank pain
MS
Arthralgia
Arthritis
Joint swelling
Myalgias
Back pain
Heme
Bleeding
Bruising
Lymph
Swelling

Endo
Polyuria
Polydypsia
Polyphagia
Derm
Rash
Pruritis
Wound(s)
Neuro
Weakness
Seizures
Parasthesias
Tremors
Syncope
Psych
Anxiety
Depression

+ ROS Findings

PE vitals HR   BP   RR   T   SPO2   Ht   Wt   BMI%

(check any)	**Neck**	**Pulm**	**Neuro**
General	( ) Midline trachea	( ) No retractions	( ) AAO x 3
( ) No Acute Distress	( ) nl thyroid w/o	( ) No dullness	( ) CN II-XII intact
( ) Cooperative	enlargement	( ) No fremitus	( ) nl sensation
( ) nl Hygiene	( ) No	( ) No wheezing/	( ) Reflexes 2+ &
Eyes	lymphadenopathy	rales/rhonchi	symmetrical
( ) nl conjunctiva	**CV**	**GI**	( ) nl memory
( ) PERRLA	( ) PMI	( ) No masses/	( ) nl speech
( ) Size___	nondisplaced	tenderness	**MSK**
( ) nl Fundus	( ) No murmur/	( ) No hep/	( ) nl tone
( ) nl Discs/vessels	gallop/rub	splenomegaly	( ) nl bulk
( ) No scleral icterus	( ) nl intensity w/o	( ) nl bowel sounds	( ) nl gait
ENT	bruit	( ) No dullness	( ) nl ROM UE
( ) No scars/masses	( ) No JVD	( ) Heme (-) stool	( ) nl ROM LE
( ) nl canals/ TM	( ) nl femoral/pedal	**GU**	L___/5 UE R___/5
( ) nl hearing bilat	pulses	( ) nl ext genitalia	L___/5 LE R___/5
( ) nl teeth/tongue	( ) No pedal	( ) No hernia	
	edema		

+ PE Findings

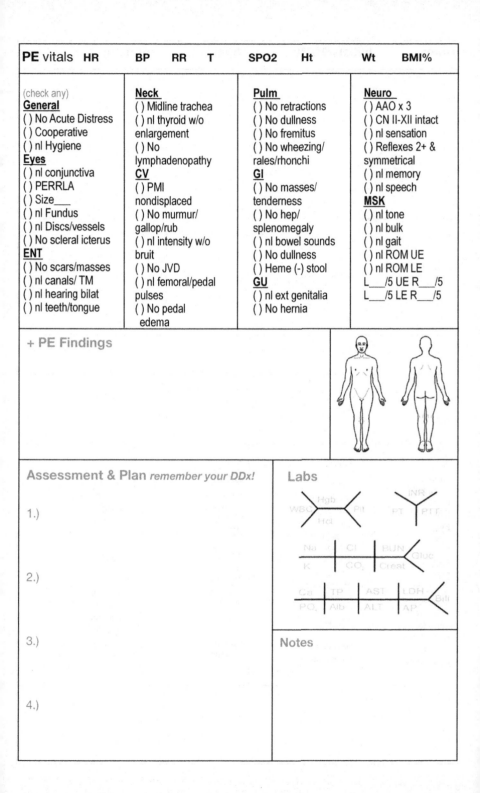

Assessment & Plan *remember your DDx!*

1.)

2.)

3.)

4.)

Labs

Notes

Date:	Initials/MRN:	Age:	Rotation:

CC: _____ y/o M/F
HPI: *symptoms/pertinent +/- ROS/prior episodes/recent travel/sick contacts*

PMHx *child/adult illness /hospitalizations/ immunizations*

SurgHx *type/when/ why/complications*

FamHx *parents/siblings/ children*

SHx *smoker/ETOH/illicits/exercise/sex/maritalstatus*

Allergies *meds/foods/ environmental/reactions*

Meds *reason/dose/time/route/compliance/vitamins/ herbs/otcs*

ROS (circle any)

Gen
Fatigue
Weight +/-
Chills
Night sweats
Eyes
Pain
Redness
Vision changes
ENT
Headache
Hoarseness
Sore throat
Sinus sx
Hearing loss
Tinnitus
Runny nose

Pulm
Cough
SOB
Wheezing
Hemoptysis
CV
Chest pain
Edema
PND
Orthopnea
Palpitations
Claudication
GI
Abd pain
N/V
Heartburn
Bloody stools

GU
Dysuria
Frequency
Hematuria
Discharge
Flank pain
MS
Arthralgia
Arthritis
Joint swelling
Myalgias
Back pain
Heme
Bleeding
Bruising
Lymph
Swelling

Endo
Polyuria
Polydypsia
Polyphagia
Derm
Rash
Pruritis
Wound(s)
Neuro
Weakness
Seizures
Parasthesias
Tremors
Syncope
Psych
Anxiety
Depression

+ ROS Findings

PE vitals HR	BP RR T	SPO2 Ht	Wt BMI%

(check any)	**Neck**	**Pulm**	**Neuro**
General	( ) Midline trachea	( ) No retractions	( ) AAO x 3
( ) No Acute Distress	( ) nl thyroid w/o	( ) No dullness	( ) CN II-XII intact
( ) Cooperative	enlargement	( ) No fremitus	( ) nl sensation
( ) nl Hygiene	( ) No	( ) No wheezing/	( ) Reflexes 2+ &
Eyes	lymphadenopathy	rales/rhonchi	symmetrical
( ) nl conjunctiva	**CV**	**GI**	( ) nl memory
( ) PERRLA	( ) PMI	( ) No masses/	( ) nl speech
( ) Size___	nondisplaced	tenderness	**MSK**
( ) nl Fundus	( ) No murmur/	( ) No hep/	( ) nl tone
( ) nl Discs/vessels	gallop/rub	splenomegaly	( ) nl bulk
( ) No scleral icterus	( ) nl intensity w/o	( ) nl bowel sounds	( ) nl gait
ENT	bruit	( ) No dullness	( ) nl ROM UE
( ) No scars/masses	( ) No JVD	( ) Heme (-) stool	( ) nl ROM LE
( ) nl canals/ TM	( ) nl femoral/pedal	**GU**	L___/5 UE R___/5
( ) nl hearing bilat	pulses	( ) nl ext genitalia	L___/5 LE R___/5
( ) nl teeth/tongue	( ) No pedal	( ) No hernia	
	edema		

+ PE Findings

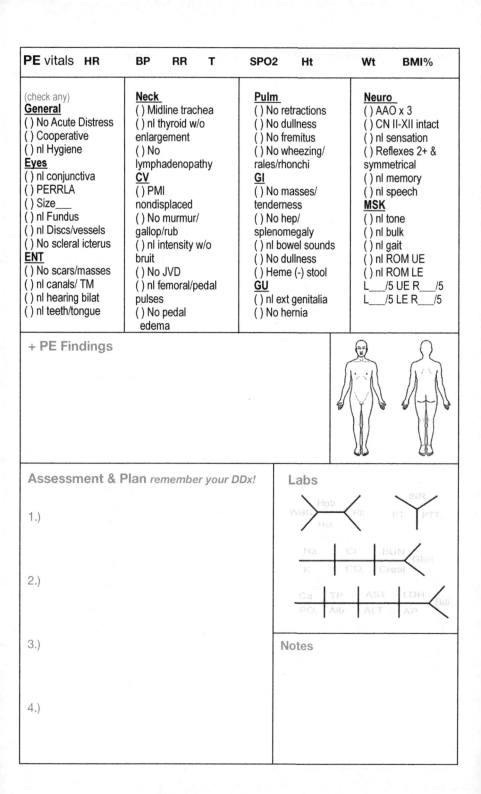

Assessment & Plan *remember your DDx!*

1.)

2.)

3.)

4.)

Labs

Hgb
WBC   Plt
Hct

INR
PT   PTT

Na   Cl   BUN   Gluc
K   CO₂   Creat

Ca   TP   AST   LDH   Bili
PO₄   Alb   ALT   AP

Notes

Date: **Initials/MRN:**   **Age:**   **Rotation:**

CC: _____ y/o M/F

HPI: *symptoms/pertinent +/- ROS/prior episodes/recent travel/sick contacts*

PMHx *child/adult illness /hospitalizations/ immunizations*

SurgHx *type/when/ why/complications*

FamHx *parents/siblings/ children*

SHx *smoker/ETOH/illicits/exercise/sex/maritalstatus*

Allergies *meds/foods/ environmental/reactions*

Meds *reason/dose/time/route/compliance/vitamins/ herbs/otcs*

ROS (circle any)

Gen	Pulm	GU	Endo
Fatigue	Cough	Dysuria	Polyuria
Weight +/-	SOB	Frequency	Polydypsia
Chills	Wheezing	Hematuria	Polyphagia
Night sweats	Hemoptysis	Discharge	**Derm**
Eyes	**CV**	Flank pain	Rash
Pain	Chest pain	**MS**	Pruritis
Redness	Edema	Arthralgia	Wound(s)
Vision changes	PND	Arthritis	**Neuro**
ENT	Orthopnea	Joint swelling	Weakness
Headache	Palpitations	Myalgias	Seizures
Hoarseness	Claudication	Back pain	Parasthesias
Sore throat	**GI**	**Heme**	Tremors
Sinus sx	Abd pain	Bleeding	Syncope
Hearing loss	N/V	Bruising	**Psych**
Tinnitus	Heartburn	**Lymph**	Anxiety
Runny nose	Bloody stools	Swelling	Depression

+ ROS Findings

PE vitals	HR	BP	RR	T	SPO2	Ht	Wt	BMI%

(check any)	**Neck**	**Pulm**	**Neuro**
General	( ) Midline trachea	( ) No retractions	( ) AAO x 3
( ) No Acute Distress	( ) nl thyroid w/o	( ) No dullness	( ) CN II-XII intact
( ) Cooperative	enlargement	( ) No fremitus	( ) nl sensation
( ) nl Hygiene	( ) No	( ) No wheezing/	( ) Reflexes 2+ &
Eyes	lymphadenopathy	rales/rhonchi	symmetrical
( ) nl conjunctiva	**CV**	**GI**	( ) nl memory
( ) PERRLA	( ) PMI	( ) No masses/	( ) nl speech
( ) Size___	nondisplaced	tenderness	**MSK**
( ) nl Fundus	( ) No murmur/	( ) No hep/	( ) nl tone
( ) nl Discs/vessels	gallop/rub	splenomegaly	( ) nl bulk
( ) No scleral icterus	( ) nl intensity w/o	( ) nl bowel sounds	( ) nl gait
ENT	bruit	( ) No dullness	( ) nl ROM UE
( ) No scars/masses	( ) No JVD	( ) Heme (-) stool	( ) nl ROM LE
( ) nl canals/ TM	( ) nl femoral/pedal	**GU**	L___/5 UE R___/5
( ) nl hearing bilat	pulses	( ) nl ext genitalia	L___/5 LE R___/5
( ) nl teeth/tongue	( ) No pedal	( ) No hernia	
	edema		

+ PE Findings

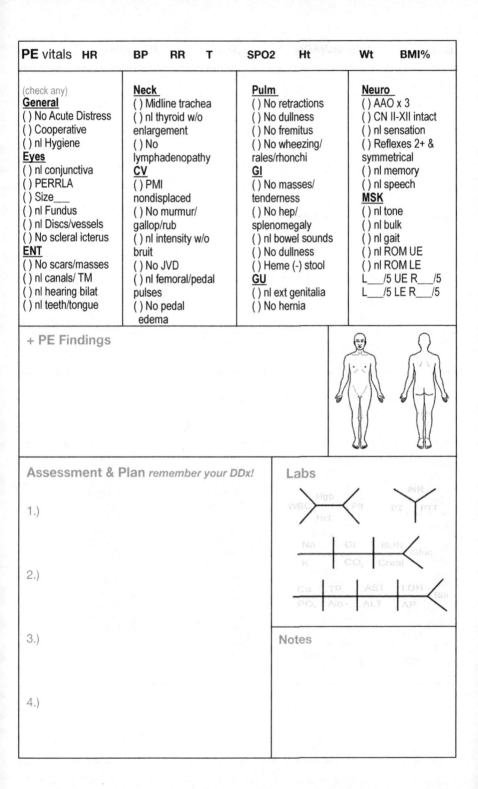

Assessment & Plan *remember your DDx!*

1.)

2.)

3.)

4.)

Labs

Notes

Date:	Initials/MRN:	Age:	Rotation:

CC: _____ y/o M/F
HPI: *symptoms/pertinent +/- ROS/prior episodes/recent travel/sick contacts*

PMHx *child/adult illness /hospitalizations/ immunizations*	**SurgHx** *type/when/ why/complications*	**FamHx** *parents/siblings/ children*

SHx *smoker/ETOH/illicits/exercise/sex/maritalstatus*

Allergies *meds/foods/ environmental/reactions*	**Meds** *reason/dose/time/route/compliance/vitamins/ herbs/otcs*

ROS (circle any)

Gen	**Pulm**	**GU**	**Endo**
Fatigue	Cough	Dysuria	Polyuria
Weight +/-	SOB	Frequency	Polydypsia
Chills	Wheezing	Hematuria	Polyphagia
Night sweats	Hemoptysis	Discharge	**Derm**
Eyes	**CV**	Flank pain	Rash
Pain	Chest pain	**MS**	Pruritis
Redness	Edema	Arthralgia	Wound(s)
Vision changes	PND	Arthritis	**Neuro**
ENT	Orthopnea	Joint swelling	Weakness
Headache	Palpitations	Myalgias	Seizures
Hoarseness	Claudication	Back pain	Parasthesias
Sore throat	**GI**	**Heme**	Tremors
Sinus sx	Abd pain	Bleeding	Syncope
Hearing loss	N/V	Bruising	**Psych**
Tinnitus	Heartburn	**Lymph**	Anxiety
Runny nose	Bloody stools	Swelling	Depression

+ ROS Findings

PE vitals **HR**   **BP**   **RR**   **T**   **SPO2**   **Ht**   **Wt**   **BMI%**

(check any)	**Neck**	**Pulm**	**Neuro**
General	( ) Midline trachea	( ) No retractions	( ) AAO x 3
( ) No Acute Distress	( ) nl thyroid w/o	( ) No dullness	( ) CN II-XII intact
( ) Cooperative	enlargement	( ) No fremitus	( ) nl sensation
( ) nl Hygiene	( ) No	( ) No wheezing/	( ) Reflexes 2+ &
Eyes	lymphadenopathy	rales/rhonchi	symmetrical
( ) nl conjunctiva	**CV**	**GI**	( ) nl memory
( ) PERRLA	( ) PMI	( ) No masses/	( ) nl speech
( ) Size___	nondisplaced	tenderness	**MSK**
( ) nl Fundus	( ) No murmur/	( ) No hep/	( ) nl tone
( ) nl Discs/vessels	gallop/rub	splenomegaly	( ) nl bulk
( ) No scleral icterus	( ) nl intensity w/o	( ) nl bowel sounds	( ) nl gait
ENT	bruit	( ) No dullness	( ) nl ROM UE
( ) No scars/masses	( ) No JVD	( ) Heme (-) stool	( ) nl ROM LE
( ) nl canals/ TM	( ) nl femoral/pedal	**GU**	L___/5 UE R___/5
( ) nl hearing bilat	pulses	( ) nl ext genitalia	L___/5 LE R___/5
( ) nl teeth/tongue	( ) No pedal	( ) No hernia	
	edema		

+ PE Findings

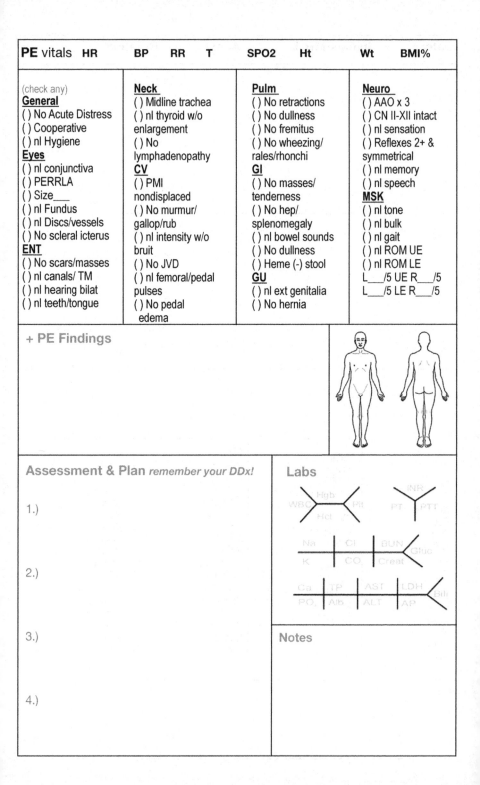

Assessment & Plan *remember your DDx!*

1.)

2.)

3.)

4.)

Labs

Hgb
WBC   Plt
Hct

INR
PT   PTT

Na   Cl   BUN
                        Gluc
K   CO₂   Creat

Ca   TP   AST   LDH
                              Bili
PO₄   Alb   ALT   AP

Notes

Date:	Initials/MRN:	Age:	Rotation:

CC: _____ y/o M/F
HPI: *symptoms/pertinent +/- ROS/prior episodes/recent travel/sick contacts*

PMHx *child/adult illness /hospitalizations/ immunizations*

SurgHx *type/when/ why/complications*

FamHx *parents/siblings/ children*

SHx *smoker/ETOH/illicits/exercise/sex/maritalstatus*

Allergies *meds/foods/ environmental/reactions*

Meds *reason/dose/time/route/compliance/vitamins/ herbs/otcs*

ROS (circle any)

Gen
Fatigue
Weight +/-
Chills
Night sweats
Eyes
Pain
Redness
Vision changes
ENT
Headache
Hoarseness
Sore throat
Sinus sx
Hearing loss
Tinnitus
Runny nose

Pulm
Cough
SOB
Wheezing
Hemoptysis
CV
Chest pain
Edema
PND
Orthopnea
Palpitations
Claudication
GI
Abd pain
N/V
Heartburn
Bloody stools

GU
Dysuria
Frequency
Hematuria
Discharge
Flank pain
MS
Arthralgia
Arthritis
Joint swelling
Myalgias
Back pain
Heme
Bleeding
Bruising
Lymph
Swelling

Endo
Polyuria
Polydypsia
Polyphagia
Derm
Rash
Pruritis
Wound(s)
Neuro
Weakness
Seizures
Parasthesias
Tremors
Syncope
Psych
Anxiety
Depression

+ ROS Findings

PE vitals	**HR**	**BP**	**RR**	**T**		**SPO2**	**Ht**		**Wt**	**BMI%**

(check any) **General** ( ) No Acute Distress ( ) Cooperative ( ) nl Hygiene **Eyes** ( ) nl conjunctiva ( ) PERRLA ( ) Size___ ( ) nl Fundus ( ) nl Discs/vessels ( ) No scleral icterus **ENT** ( ) No scars/masses ( ) nl canals/ TM ( ) nl hearing bilat ( ) nl teeth/tongue	**Neck** ( ) Midline trachea ( ) nl thyroid w/o enlargement ( ) No lymphadenopathy **CV** ( ) PMI nondisplaced ( ) No murmur/ gallop/rub ( ) nl intensity w/o bruit ( ) No JVD ( ) nl femoral/pedal pulses ( ) No pedal edema	**Pulm** ( ) No retractions ( ) No dullness ( ) No fremitus ( ) No wheezing/ rales/rhonchi **GI** ( ) No masses/ tenderness ( ) No hep/ splenomegaly ( ) nl bowel sounds ( ) No dullness ( ) Heme (-) stool **GU** ( ) nl ext genitalia ( ) No hernia	**Neuro** ( ) AAO x 3 ( ) CN II-XII intact ( ) nl sensation ( ) Reflexes 2+ & symmetrical ( ) nl memory ( ) nl speech **MSK** ( ) nl tone ( ) nl bulk ( ) nl gait ( ) nl ROM UE ( ) nl ROM LE L___/5 UE R___/5 L___/5 LE R___/5

+ PE Findings

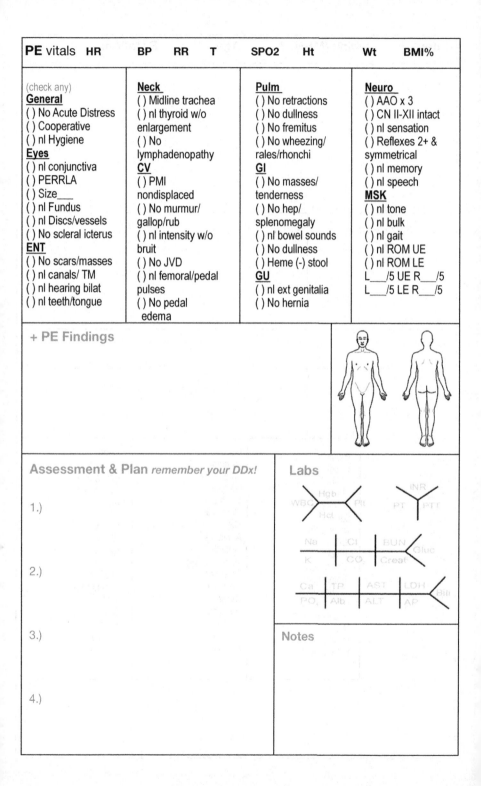

Assessment & Plan *remember your DDx!*

1.)

2.)

3.)

4.)

Labs

Notes

Date: **Initials/MRN:**   **Age:**   **Rotation:**

CC: _____ y/o M/F
HPI: *symptoms/pertinent +/- ROS/prior episodes/recent travel/sick contacts*

PMHx *child/adult illness /hospitalizations/ immunizations*

SurgHx *type/when/ why/complications*

FamHx *parents/siblings/ children*

SHx *smoker/ETOH/illicits/exercise/sex/maritalstatus*

Allergies *meds/foods/ environmental/reactions*

Meds *reason/dose/time/route/compliance/vitamins/ herbs/otcs*

ROS (circle any)

Gen
Fatigue
Weight +/-
Chills
Night sweats
Eyes
Pain
Redness
Vision changes
ENT
Headache
Hoarseness
Sore throat
Sinus sx
Hearing loss
Tinnitus
Runny nose

Pulm
Cough
SOB
Wheezing
Hemoptysis
CV
Chest pain
Edema
PND
Orthopnea
Palpitations
Claudication
GI
Abd pain
N/V
Heartburn
Bloody stools

GU
Dysuria
Frequency
Hematuria
Discharge
Flank pain
MS
Arthralgia
Arthritis
Joint swelling
Myalgias
Back pain
Heme
Bleeding
Bruising
Lymph
Swelling

Endo
Polyuria
Polydypsia
Polyphagia
Derm
Rash
Pruritis
Wound(s)
Neuro
Weakness
Seizures
Parasthesias
Tremors
Syncope
Psych
Anxiety
Depression

+ ROS Findings

PE vitals **HR**   **BP** **RR** **T**   **SPO2** **Ht**   **Wt** **BMI%**

(check any)	**Neck**	**Pulm**	**Neuro**
General	( ) Midline trachea	( ) No retractions	( ) AAO x 3
( ) No Acute Distress	( ) nl thyroid w/o	( ) No dullness	( ) CN II-XII intact
( ) Cooperative	enlargement	( ) No fremitus	( ) nl sensation
( ) nl Hygiene	( ) No	( ) No wheezing/	( ) Reflexes 2+ &
Eyes	lymphadenopathy	rales/rhonchi	symmetrical
( ) nl conjunctiva	**CV**	**GI**	( ) nl memory
( ) PERRLA	( ) PMI	( ) No masses/	( ) nl speech
( ) Size___	nondisplaced	tenderness	**MSK**
( ) nl Fundus	( ) No murmur/	( ) No hep/	( ) nl tone
( ) nl Discs/vessels	gallop/rub	splenomegaly	( ) nl bulk
( ) No scleral icterus	( ) nl intensity w/o	( ) nl bowel sounds	( ) nl gait
ENT	bruit	( ) No dullness	( ) nl ROM UE
( ) No scars/masses	( ) No JVD	( ) Heme (-) stool	( ) nl ROM LE
( ) nl canals/ TM	( ) nl femoral/pedal	**GU**	L___/5 UE R___/5
( ) nl hearing bilat	pulses	( ) nl ext genitalia	L___/5 LE R___/5
( ) nl teeth/tongue	( ) No pedal	( ) No hernia	
	edema		

+ PE Findings

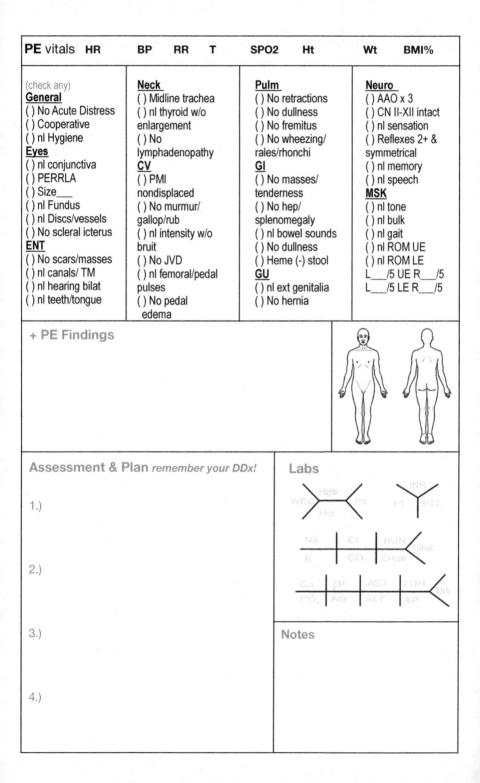

Assessment & Plan *remember your DDx!*

1.)

2.)

3.)

4.)

Labs

Notes

Date:	Initials/MRN:	Age:	Rotation:

CC: _____ y/o M/F
HPI: *symptoms/pertinent +/- ROS/prior episodes/recent travel/sick contacts*

PMHx *child/adult illness /hospitalizations/ immunizations*	**SurgHx** *type/when/ why/complications*	**FamHx** *parents/siblings/ children*

SHx *smoker/ETOH/illicits/exercise/sex/maritalstatus*

Allergies *meds/foods/ environmental/reactions*	**Meds** *reason/dose/time/route/compliance/vitamins/ herbs/otcs*

ROS (circle any)

Gen	**Pulm**	**GU**	**Endo**
Fatigue	Cough	Dysuria	Polyuria
Weight +/-	SOB	Frequency	Polydypsia
Chills	Wheezing	Hematuria	Polyphagia
Night sweats	Hemoptysis	Discharge	**Derm**
Eyes	**CV**	Flank pain	Rash
Pain	Chest pain	**MS**	Pruritis
Redness	Edema	Arthralgia	Wound(s)
Vision changes	PND	Arthritis	**Neuro**
ENT	Orthopnea	Joint swelling	Weakness
Headache	Palpitations	Myalgias	Seizures
Hoarseness	Claudication	Back pain	Parasthesias
Sore throat	**GI**	**Heme**	Tremors
Sinus sx	Abd pain	Bleeding	Syncope
Hearing loss	N/V	Bruising	**Psych**
Tinnitus	Heartburn	**Lymph**	Anxiety
Runny nose	Bloody stools	Swelling	Depression

+ ROS Findings

PE vitals	**HR**	**BP**	**RR**	**T**	**SPO2**	**Ht**	**Wt**	**BMI%**

(check any)

General
( ) No Acute Distress
( ) Cooperative
( ) nl Hygiene

Eyes
( ) nl conjunctiva
( ) PERRLA
( ) Size___
( ) nl Fundus
( ) nl Discs/vessels
( ) No scleral icterus

ENT
( ) No scars/masses
( ) nl canals/ TM
( ) nl hearing bilat
( ) nl teeth/tongue

Neck
( ) Midline trachea
( ) nl thyroid w/o enlargement
( ) No lymphadenopathy

CV
( ) PMI nondisplaced
( ) No murmur/ gallop/rub
( ) nl intensity w/o bruit
( ) No JVD
( ) nl femoral/pedal pulses
( ) No pedal edema

Pulm
( ) No retractions
( ) No dullness
( ) No fremitus
( ) No wheezing/ rales/rhonchi

GI
( ) No masses/ tenderness
( ) No hep/ splenomegaly
( ) nl bowel sounds
( ) No dullness
( ) Heme (-) stool

GU
( ) nl ext genitalia
( ) No hernia

Neuro
( ) AAO x 3
( ) CN II-XII intact
( ) nl sensation
( ) Reflexes 2+ & symmetrical
( ) nl memory
( ) nl speech

MSK
( ) nl tone
( ) nl bulk
( ) nl gait
( ) nl ROM UE
( ) nl ROM LE
L___/5 UE R___/5
L___/5 LE R___/5

+ PE Findings

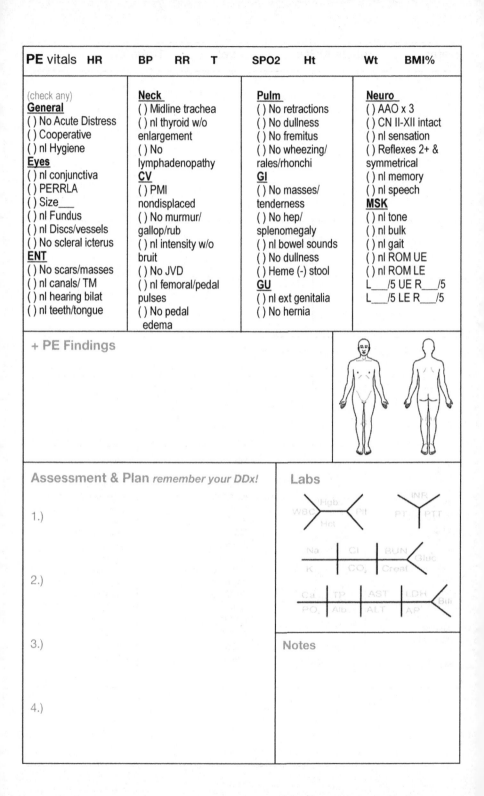

Assessment & Plan *remember your DDx!*

1.)

2.)

3.)

4.)

Labs

Notes

Date:	Initials/MRN:	Age:	Rotation:

CC: _____ y/o M/F
HPI: *symptoms/pertinent +/- ROS/prior episodes/recent travel/sick contacts*

PMHx *child/adult illness /hospitalizations/ immunizations*

SurgHx *type/when/ why/complications*

FamHx *parents/siblings/ children*

SHx *smoker/ETOH/illicits/exercise/sex/maritalstatus*

Allergies *meds/foods/ environmental/reactions*

Meds *reason/dose/time/route/compliance/vitamins/ herbs/otcs*

ROS (circle any)

Gen
Fatigue
Weight +/-
Chills
Night sweats
Eyes
Pain
Redness
Vision changes
ENT
Headache
Hoarseness
Sore throat
Sinus sx
Hearing loss
Tinnitus
Runny nose

Pulm
Cough
SOB
Wheezing
Hemoptysis
CV
Chest pain
Edema
PND
Orthopnea
Palpitations
Claudication
GI
Abd pain
N/V
Heartburn
Bloody stools

GU
Dysuria
Frequency
Hematuria
Discharge
Flank pain
MS
Arthralgia
Arthritis
Joint swelling
Myalgias
Back pain
Heme
Bleeding
Bruising
Lymph
Swelling

Endo
Polyuria
Polydypsia
Polyphagia
Derm
Rash
Pruritis
Wound(s)
Neuro
Weakness
Seizures
Parasthesias
Tremors
Syncope
Psych
Anxiety
Depression

+ ROS Findings

| **PE** vitals | HR | BP | RR | T | SPO2 | Ht | Wt | BMI% |

(check any)	**Neck**	**Pulm**	**Neuro**
General	( ) Midline trachea	( ) No retractions	( ) AAO x 3
( ) No Acute Distress	( ) nl thyroid w/o	( ) No dullness	( ) CN II-XII intact
( ) Cooperative	enlargement	( ) No fremitus	( ) nl sensation
( ) nl Hygiene	( ) No	( ) No wheezing/	( ) Reflexes 2+ &
Eyes	lymphadenopathy	rales/rhonchi	symmetrical
( ) nl conjunctiva	**CV**	**GI**	( ) nl memory
( ) PERRLA	( ) PMI	( ) No masses/	( ) nl speech
( ) Size___	nondisplaced	tenderness	**MSK**
( ) nl Fundus	( ) No murmur/	( ) No hep/	( ) nl tone
( ) nl Discs/vessels	gallop/rub	splenomegaly	( ) nl bulk
( ) No scleral icterus	( ) nl intensity w/o	( ) nl bowel sounds	( ) nl gait
ENT	bruit	( ) No dullness	( ) nl ROM UE
( ) No scars/masses	( ) No JVD	( ) Heme (-) stool	( ) nl ROM LE
( ) nl canals/ TM	( ) nl femoral/pedal	**GU**	L___/5 UE R___/5
( ) nl hearing bilat	pulses	( ) nl ext genitalia	L___/5 LE R___/5
( ) nl teeth/tongue	( ) No pedal	( ) No hernia	
	edema		

+ PE Findings

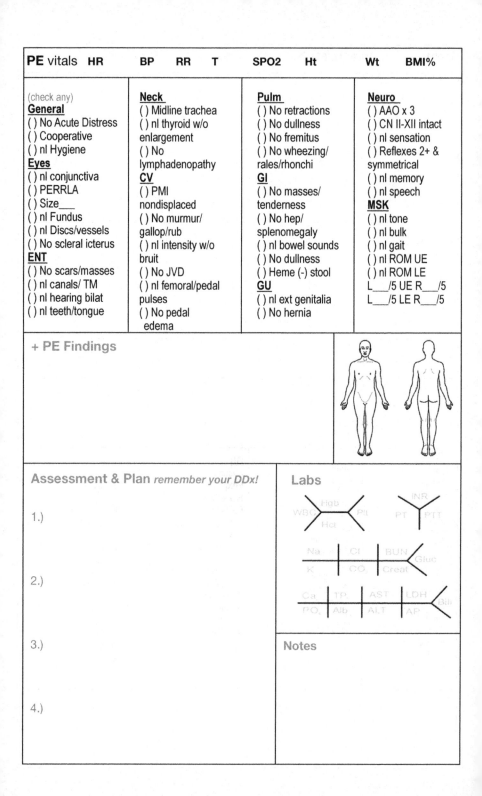

Assessment & Plan *remember your DDx!*

1.)

2.)

3.)

4.)

Labs

Notes

Date:	Initials/MRN:	Age:	Rotation:

CC: _____ y/o M/F
HPI: *symptoms/pertinent +/- ROS/prior episodes/recent travel/sick contacts*

PMHx *child/adult illness /hospitalizations/ immunizations*	**SurgHx** *type/when/ why/complications*	**FamHx** *parents/siblings/ children*

SHx *smoker/ETOH/illicits/exercise/sex/maritalstatus*

Allergies *meds/foods/ environmental/reactions*	**Meds** *reason/dose/time/route/compliance/vitamins/ herbs/otcs*

ROS (circle any)

Gen	**Pulm**	**GU**	**Endo**
Fatigue	Cough	Dysuria	Polyuria
Weight +/-	SOB	Frequency	Polydypsia
Chills	Wheezing	Hematuria	Polyphagia
Night sweats	Hemoptysis	Discharge	**Derm**
Eyes	**CV**	Flank pain	Rash
Pain	Chest pain	**MS**	Pruritis
Redness	Edema	Arthralgia	Wound(s)
Vision changes	PND	Arthritis	**Neuro**
ENT	Orthopnea	Joint swelling	Weakness
Headache	Palpitations	Myalgias	Seizures
Hoarseness	Claudication	Back pain	Parasthesias
Sore throat	**GI**	**Heme**	Tremors
Sinus sx	Abd pain	Bleeding	Syncope
Hearing loss	N/V	Bruising	**Psych**
Tinnitus	Heartburn	**Lymph**	Anxiety
Runny nose	Bloody stools	Swelling	Depression

+ ROS Findings

PE vitals	HR	BP	RR	T	SPO2	Ht	Wt	BMI%

(check any) **General**	**Neck**	**Pulm**	**Neuro**
( ) No Acute Distress	( ) Midline trachea	( ) No retractions	( ) AAO x 3
( ) Cooperative	( ) nl thyroid w/o	( ) No dullness	( ) CN II-XII intact
( ) nl Hygiene	enlargement	( ) No fremitus	( ) nl sensation
Eyes	( ) No	( ) No wheezing/	( ) Reflexes 2+ &
( ) nl conjunctiva	lymphadenopathy	rales/rhonchi	symmetrical
( ) PERRLA	**CV**	**GI**	( ) nl memory
( ) Size___	( ) PMI	( ) No masses/	( ) nl speech
( ) nl Fundus	nondisplaced	tenderness	**MSK**
( ) nl Discs/vessels	( ) No murmur/	( ) No hep/	( ) nl tone
( ) No scleral icterus	gallop/rub	splenomegaly	( ) nl bulk
ENT	( ) nl intensity w/o	( ) nl bowel sounds	( ) nl gait
( ) No scars/masses	bruit	( ) No dullness	( ) nl ROM UE
( ) nl canals/ TM	( ) No JVD	( ) Heme (-) stool	( ) nl ROM LE
( ) nl hearing bilat	( ) nl femoral/pedal	**GU**	L___/5 UE R___/5
( ) nl teeth/tongue	pulses	( ) nl ext genitalia	L___/5 LE R___/5
	( ) No pedal	( ) No hernia	
	edema		

+ PE Findings

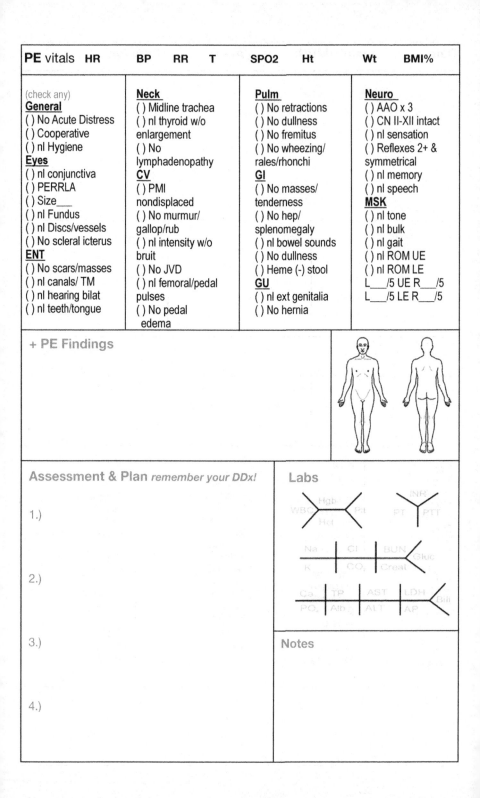

Assessment & Plan *remember your DDx!*

1.)

2.)

3.)

4.)

Labs

Notes

Date:	Initials/MRN:	Age:	Rotation:

CC: _____ y/o M/F
HPI: *symptoms/pertinent +/- ROS/prior episodes/recent travel/sick contacts*

PMHx *child/adult illness /hospitalizations/ immunizations*	**SurgHx** *type/when/ why/complications*	**FamHx** *parents/siblings/ children*

SHx *smoker/ETOH/illicits/exercise/sex/maritalstatus*

Allergies *meds/foods/ environmental/reactions*	**Meds** *reason/dose/time/route/compliance/vitamins/ herbs/otcs*

ROS (circle any)

Gen	**Pulm**	**GU**	**Endo**
Fatigue	Cough	Dysuria	Polyuria
Weight +/-	SOB	Frequency	Polydypsia
Chills	Wheezing	Hematuria	Polyphagia
Night sweats	Hemoptysis	Discharge	**Derm**
Eyes	**CV**	Flank pain	Rash
Pain	Chest pain	**MS**	Pruritis
Redness	Edema	Arthralgia	Wound(s)
Vision changes	PND	Arthritis	**Neuro**
ENT	Orthopnea	Joint swelling	Weakness
Headache	Palpitations	Myalgias	Seizures
Hoarseness	Claudication	Back pain	Parasthesias
Sore throat	**GI**	**Heme**	Tremors
Sinus sx	Abd pain	Bleeding	Syncope
Hearing loss	N/V	Bruising	**Psych**
Tinnitus	Heartburn	**Lymph**	Anxiety
Runny nose	Bloody stools	Swelling	Depression

+ ROS Findings

PE vitals	**HR**	**BP**	**RR**	**T**	**SPO2**	**Ht**	**Wt**	**BMI%**

(check any)

General	**Neck**	**Pulm**	**Neuro**
( ) No Acute Distress	( ) Midline trachea	( ) No retractions	( ) AAO x 3
( ) Cooperative	( ) nl thyroid w/o	( ) No dullness	( ) CN II-XII intact
( ) nl Hygiene	enlargement	( ) No fremitus	( ) nl sensation
Eyes	( ) No	( ) No wheezing/	( ) Reflexes 2+ &
( ) nl conjunctiva	lymphadenopathy	rales/rhonchi	symmetrical
( ) PERRLA	**CV**	**GI**	( ) nl memory
( ) Size___	( ) PMI	( ) No masses/	( ) nl speech
( ) nl Fundus	nondisplaced	tenderness	**MSK**
( ) nl Discs/vessels	( ) No murmur/	( ) No hep/	( ) nl tone
( ) No scleral icterus	gallop/rub	splenomegaly	( ) nl bulk
ENT	( ) nl intensity w/o	( ) nl bowel sounds	( ) nl gait
( ) No scars/masses	bruit	( ) No dullness	( ) nl ROM UE
( ) nl canals/ TM	( ) No JVD	( ) Heme (-) stool	( ) nl ROM LE
( ) nl hearing bilat	( ) nl femoral/pedal	**GU**	L___/5 UE R___/5
( ) nl teeth/tongue	pulses	( ) nl ext genitalia	L___/5 LE R___/5
	( ) No pedal	( ) No hernia	
	edema		

+ PE Findings

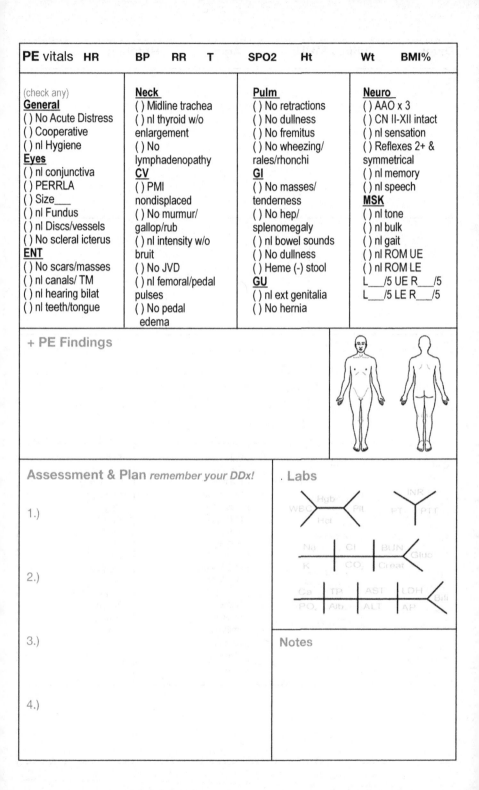

Assessment & Plan *remember your DDx!*

1.)

2.)

3.)

4.)

. Labs

Hgb
WBC — Plt
Hct

INR
PT — PTT

Na | Cl | BUN
K | CO₂ | Creat — Gluc

Ca | TP | AST | LDH
PO₄ | Alb | ALT | AP — Bili

Notes

Date:	Initials/MRN:	Age:	Rotation:

CC: _____ y/o M/F
HPI: *symptoms/pertinent +/- ROS/prior episodes/recent travel/sick contacts*

PMHx *child/adult illness /hospitalizations/ immunizations*	**SurgHx** *type/when/ why/complications*	**FamHx** *parents/siblings/ children*

SHx *smoker/ETOH/illicits/exercise/sex/maritalstatus*

Allergies *meds/foods/ environmental/reactions*	**Meds** *reason/dose/time/route/compliance/vitamins/ herbs/otcs*

ROS (circle any)

Gen	**Pulm**	**GU**	**Endo**
Fatigue	Cough	Dysuria	Polyuria
Weight +/-	SOB	Frequency	Polydypsia
Chills	Wheezing	Hematuria	Polyphagia
Night sweats	Hemoptysis	Discharge	**Derm**
Eyes	**CV**	Flank pain	Rash
Pain	Chest pain	**MS**	Pruritis
Redness	Edema	Arthralgia	Wound(s)
Vision changes	PND	Arthritis	**Neuro**
ENT	Orthopnea	Joint swelling	Weakness
Headache	Palpitations	Myalgias	Seizures
Hoarseness	Claudication	Back pain	Parasthesias
Sore throat	**GI**	**Heme**	Tremors
Sinus sx	Abd pain	Bleeding	Syncope
Hearing loss	N/V	Bruising	**Psych**
Tinnitus	Heartburn	**Lymph**	Anxiety
Runny nose	Bloody stools	Swelling	Depression

+ ROS Findings

PE vitals	HR	BP	RR	T	SPO2	Ht	Wt	BMI%

(check any) **General** ( ) No Acute Distress ( ) Cooperative ( ) nl Hygiene **Eyes** ( ) nl conjunctiva ( ) PERRLA ( ) Size___ ( ) nl Fundus ( ) nl Discs/vessels ( ) No scleral icterus **ENT** ( ) No scars/masses ( ) nl canals/ TM ( ) nl hearing bilat ( ) nl teeth/tongue	**Neck** ( ) Midline trachea ( ) nl thyroid w/o enlargement ( ) No lymphadenopathy **CV** ( ) PMI nondisplaced ( ) No murmur/ gallop/rub ( ) nl intensity w/o bruit ( ) No JVD ( ) nl femoral/pedal pulses ( ) No pedal edema	**Pulm** ( ) No retractions ( ) No dullness ( ) No fremitus ( ) No wheezing/ rales/rhonchi **GI** ( ) No masses/ tenderness ( ) No hep/ splenomegaly ( ) nl bowel sounds ( ) No dullness ( ) Heme (-) stool **GU** ( ) nl ext genitalia ( ) No hernia	**Neuro** ( ) AAO x 3 ( ) CN II-XII intact ( ) nl sensation ( ) Reflexes 2+ & symmetrical ( ) nl memory ( ) nl speech **MSK** ( ) nl tone ( ) nl bulk ( ) nl gait ( ) nl ROM UE ( ) nl ROM LE L___/5 UE R___/5 L___/5 LE R___/5

+ PE Findings

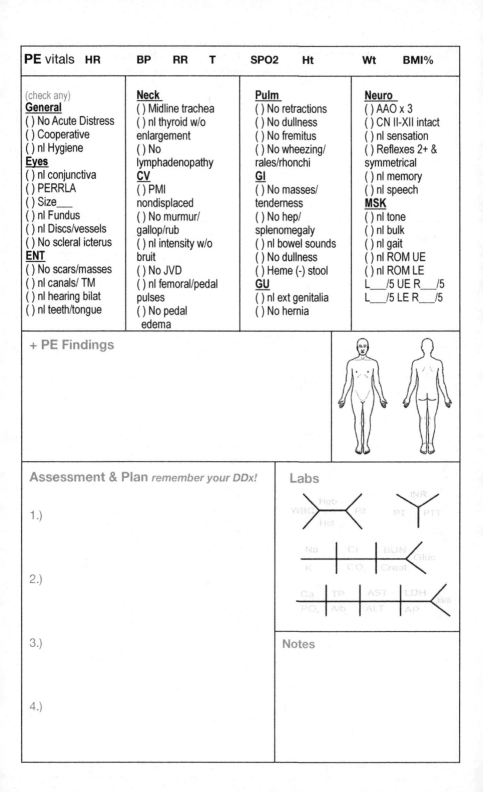

Assessment & Plan *remember your DDx!*

Labs

1.)

2.)

3.)

Notes

4.)

| **Date:** | **Initials/MRN:** | **Age:** | **Rotation:** |

CC: _____ y/o M/F
HPI: *symptoms/pertinent +/- ROS/prior episodes/recent travel/sick contacts*

PMHx *child/adult illness /hospitalizations/ immunizations*

SurgHx *type/when/ why/complications*

FamHx *parents/siblings/ children*

SHx *smoker/ETOH/illicits/exercise/sex/maritalstatus*

Allergies *meds/foods/ environmental/reactions*

Meds *reason/dose/time/route/compliance/vitamins/ herbs/otcs*

ROS (circle any)

Gen	**Pulm**	**GU**	**Endo**
Fatigue	Cough	Dysuria	Polyuria
Weight +/-	SOB	Frequency	Polydypsia
Chills	Wheezing	Hematuria	Polyphagia
Night sweats	Hemoptysis	Discharge	**Derm**
Eyes	**CV**	Flank pain	Rash
Pain	Chest pain	**MS**	Pruritis
Redness	Edema	Arthralgia	Wound(s)
Vision changes	PND	Arthritis	**Neuro**
ENT	Orthopnea	Joint swelling	Weakness
Headache	Palpitations	Myalgias	Seizures
Hoarseness	Claudication	Back pain	Parasthesias
Sore throat	**GI**	**Heme**	Tremors
Sinus sx	Abd pain	Bleeding	Syncope
Hearing loss	N/V	Bruising	**Psych**
Tinnitus	Heartburn	**Lymph**	Anxiety
Runny nose	Bloody stools	Swelling	Depression

+ ROS Findings

PE vitals	HR	BP	RR	T	SPO2	Ht	Wt	BMI%

(check any)

General
( ) No Acute Distress
( ) Cooperative
( ) nl Hygiene
Eyes
( ) nl conjunctiva
( ) PERRLA
( ) Size___
( ) nl Fundus
( ) nl Discs/vessels
( ) No scleral icterus
ENT
( ) No scars/masses
( ) nl canals/ TM
( ) nl hearing bilat
( ) nl teeth/tongue

Neck
( ) Midline trachea
( ) nl thyroid w/o
enlargement
( ) No
lymphadenopathy
CV
( ) PMI
nondisplaced
( ) No murmur/
gallop/rub
( ) nl intensity w/o
bruit
( ) No JVD
( ) nl femoral/pedal
pulses
( ) No pedal
edema

Pulm
( ) No retractions
( ) No dullness
( ) No fremitus
( ) No wheezing/
rales/rhonchi
GI
( ) No masses/
tenderness
( ) No hep/
splenomegaly
( ) nl bowel sounds
( ) No dullness
( ) Heme (-) stool
GU
( ) nl ext genitalia
( ) No hernia

Neuro
( ) AAO x 3
( ) CN II-XII intact
( ) nl sensation
( ) Reflexes 2+ &
symmetrical
( ) nl memory
( ) nl speech
MSK
( ) nl tone
( ) nl bulk
( ) nl gait
( ) nl ROM UE
( ) nl ROM LE
L___/5 UE R___/5
L___/5 LE R___/5

+ PE Findings

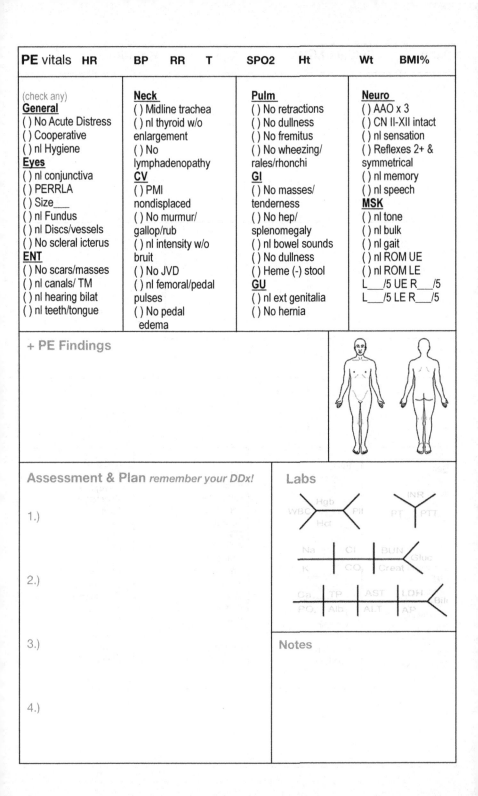

Assessment & Plan *remember your DDx!*

1.)

2.)

3.)

4.)

Labs

Notes

Date:	Initials/MRN:	Age:	Rotation:

CC: _____ y/o M/F
HPI: *symptoms/pertinent +/- ROS/prior episodes/recent travel/sick contacts*

PMHx *child/adult illness /hospitalizations/ immunizations*

SurgHx *type/when/ why/complications*

FamHx *parents/siblings/ children*

SHx *smoker/ETOH/illicits/exercise/sex/maritalstatus*

Allergies *meds/foods/ environmental/reactions*

Meds *reason/dose/time/route/compliance/vitamins/ herbs/otcs*

ROS (circle any)

Gen
Fatigue
Weight +/-
Chills
Night sweats
Eyes
Pain
Redness
Vision changes
ENT
Headache
Hoarseness
Sore throat
Sinus sx
Hearing loss
Tinnitus
Runny nose

Pulm
Cough
SOB
Wheezing
Hemoptysis
CV
Chest pain
Edema
PND
Orthopnea
Palpitations
Claudication
GI
Abd pain
N/V
Heartburn
Bloody stools

GU
Dysuria
Frequency
Hematuria
Discharge
Flank pain
MS
Arthralgia
Arthritis
Joint swelling
Myalgias
Back pain
Heme
Bleeding
Bruising
Lymph
Swelling

Endo
Polyuria
Polydypsia
Polyphagia
Derm
Rash
Pruritis
Wound(s)
Neuro
Weakness
Seizures
Parasthesias
Tremors
Syncope
Psych
Anxiety
Depression

+ ROS Findings

PE vitals   HR   BP   RR   T   SPO2   Ht   Wt   BMI%

(check any)	**Neck**	**Pulm**	**Neuro**
General	( ) Midline trachea	( ) No retractions	( ) AAO x 3
( ) No Acute Distress	( ) nl thyroid w/o	( ) No dullness	( ) CN II-XII intact
( ) Cooperative	enlargement	( ) No fremitus	( ) nl sensation
( ) nl Hygiene	( ) No	( ) No wheezing/	( ) Reflexes 2+ &
Eyes	lymphadenopathy	rales/rhonchi	symmetrical
( ) nl conjunctiva	**CV**	**GI**	( ) nl memory
( ) PERRLA	( ) PMI	( ) No masses/	( ) nl speech
( ) Size___	nondisplaced	tenderness	**MSK**
( ) nl Fundus	( ) No murmur/	( ) No hep/	( ) nl tone
( ) nl Discs/vessels	gallop/rub	splenomegaly	( ) nl bulk
( ) No scleral icterus	( ) nl intensity w/o	( ) nl bowel sounds	( ) nl gait
ENT	bruit	( ) No dullness	( ) nl ROM UE
( ) No scars/masses	( ) No JVD	( ) Heme (-) stool	( ) nl ROM LE
( ) nl canals/ TM	( ) nl femoral/pedal	**GU**	L___/5 UE R___/5
( ) nl hearing bilat	pulses	( ) nl ext genitalia	L___/5 LE R___/5
( ) nl teeth/tongue	( ) No pedal	( ) No hernia	
	edema		

+ PE Findings

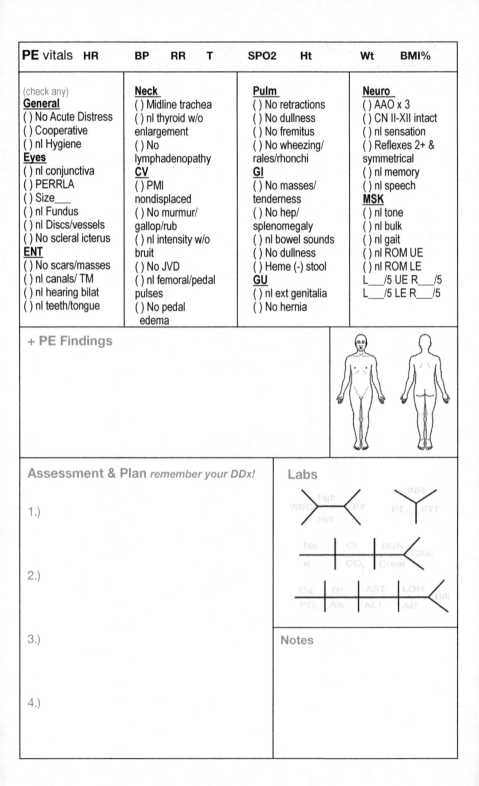

Assessment & Plan *remember your DDx!*

1.)

2.)

3.)

4.)

Labs

Hgb
WBC — Plt
Hct

INR
PT — PTT

Na | Cl | BUN
K | CO₂ | Creat — Gluc

Ca | TP | AST | LDH
PO₄ | Alb | ALT | AP — Bili

Notes

Date:	Initials/MRN:	Age:	Rotation:

CC: _____ y/o M/F
HPI: *symptoms/pertinent +/- ROS/prior episodes/recent travel/sick contacts*

PMHx *child/adult illness /hospitalizations/ immunizations*	**SurgHx** *type/when/ why/complications*	**FamHx** *parents/siblings/ children*

SHx *smoker/ETOH/illicits/exercise/sex/maritalstatus*

Allergies *meds/foods/ environmental/reactions*	**Meds** *reason/dose/time/route/compliance/vitamins/ herbs/otcs*

ROS (circle any)

Gen	**Pulm**	**GU**	**Endo**
Fatigue	Cough	Dysuria	Polyuria
Weight +/-	SOB	Frequency	Polydypsia
Chills	Wheezing	Hematuria	Polyphagia
Night sweats	Hemoptysis	Discharge	**Derm**
Eyes	**CV**	Flank pain	Rash
Pain	Chest pain	**MS**	Pruritis
Redness	Edema	Arthralgia	Wound(s)
Vision changes	PND	Arthritis	**Neuro**
ENT	Orthopnea	Joint swelling	Weakness
Headache	Palpitations	Myalgias	Seizures
Hoarseness	Claudication	Back pain	Parasthesias
Sore throat	**GI**	**Heme**	Tremors
Sinus sx	Abd pain	Bleeding	Syncope
Hearing loss	N/V	Bruising	**Psych**
Tinnitus	Heartburn	**Lymph**	Anxiety
Runny nose	Bloody stools	Swelling	Depression

+ ROS Findings

PE vitals	HR	BP	RR	T	SPO2	Ht	Wt	BMI%

(check any) **General**	**Neck**	**Pulm**	**Neuro**
( ) No Acute Distress	( ) Midline trachea	( ) No retractions	( ) AAO x 3
( ) Cooperative	( ) nl thyroid w/o	( ) No dullness	( ) CN II-XII intact
( ) nl Hygiene	enlargement	( ) No fremitus	( ) nl sensation
Eyes	( ) No	( ) No wheezing/	( ) Reflexes 2+ &
( ) nl conjunctiva	lymphadenopathy	rales/rhonchi	symmetrical
( ) PERRLA	**CV**	**GI**	( ) nl memory
( ) Size___	( ) PMI	( ) No masses/	( ) nl speech
( ) nl Fundus	nondisplaced	tenderness	**MSK**
( ) nl Discs/vessels	( ) No murmur/	( ) No hep/	( ) nl tone
( ) No scleral icterus	gallop/rub	splenomegaly	( ) nl bulk
ENT	( ) nl intensity w/o	( ) nl bowel sounds	( ) nl gait
( ) No scars/masses	bruit	( ) No dullness	( ) nl ROM UE
( ) nl canals/ TM	( ) No JVD	( ) Heme (-) stool	( ) nl ROM LE
( ) nl hearing bilat	( ) nl femoral/pedal	**GU**	L___/5 UE R___/5
( ) nl teeth/tongue	pulses	( ) nl ext genitalia	L___/5 LE R___/5
	( ) No pedal	( ) No hernia	
	edema		

+ PE Findings

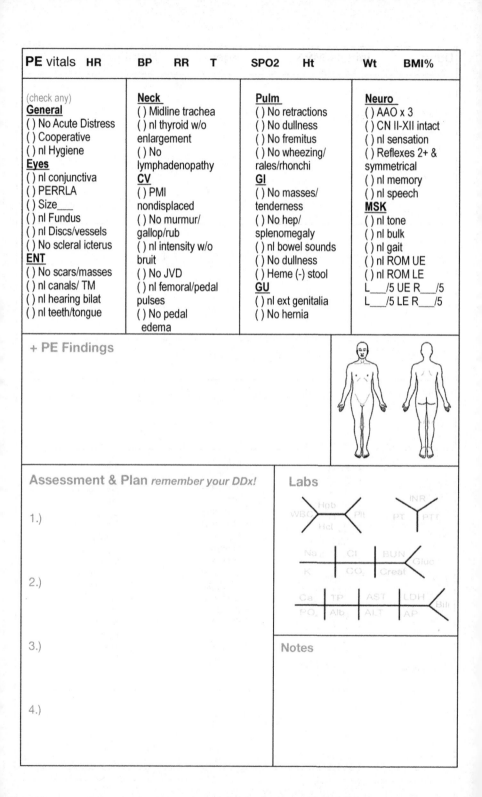

Assessment & Plan *remember your DDx!*

1.)

2.)

3.)

4.)

Labs

Notes

Date:	Initials/MRN:	Age:	Rotation:

CC: _____ y/o M/F
HPI: *symptoms/pertinent +/- ROS/prior episodes/recent travel/sick contacts*

PMHx *child/adult illness /hospitalizations/ immunizations*

SurgHx *type/when/ why/complications*

FamHx *parents/siblings/ children*

SHx *smoker/ETOH/illicits/exercise/sex/maritalstatus*

Allergies *meds/foods/ environmental/reactions*

Meds *reason/dose/time/route/compliance/vitamins/ herbs/otcs*

ROS (circle any)

Gen
Fatigue
Weight +/-
Chills
Night sweats
Eyes
Pain
Redness
Vision changes
ENT
Headache
Hoarseness
Sore throat
Sinus sx
Hearing loss
Tinnitus
Runny nose

Pulm
Cough
SOB
Wheezing
Hemoptysis
CV
Chest pain
Edema
PND
Orthopnea
Palpitations
Claudication
GI
Abd pain
N/V
Heartburn
Bloody stools

GU
Dysuria
Frequency
Hematuria
Discharge
Flank pain
MS
Arthralgia
Arthritis
Joint swelling
Myalgias
Back pain
Heme
Bleeding
Bruising
Lymph
Swelling

Endo
Polyuria
Polydypsia
Polyphagia
Derm
Rash
Pruritis
Wound(s)
Neuro
Weakness
Seizures
Parasthesias
Tremors
Syncope
Psych
Anxiety
Depression

+ ROS Findings

PE vitals HR	BP RR T	SPO2 Ht	Wt BMI%

(check any)	**Neck**	**Pulm**	**Neuro**
General	( ) Midline trachea	( ) No retractions	( ) AAO x 3
( ) No Acute Distress	( ) nl thyroid w/o	( ) No dullness	( ) CN II-XII intact
( ) Cooperative	enlargement	( ) No fremitus	( ) nl sensation
( ) nl Hygiene	( ) No	( ) No wheezing/	( ) Reflexes 2+ &
Eyes	lymphadenopathy	rales/rhonchi	symmetrical
( ) nl conjunctiva	**CV**	**GI**	( ) nl memory
( ) PERRLA	( ) PMI	( ) No masses/	( ) nl speech
( ) Size___	nondisplaced	tenderness	**MSK**
( ) nl Fundus	( ) No murmur/	( ) No hep/	( ) nl tone
( ) nl Discs/vessels	gallop/rub	splenomegaly	( ) nl bulk
( ) No scleral icterus	( ) nl intensity w/o	( ) nl bowel sounds	( ) nl gait
ENT	bruit	( ) No dullness	( ) nl ROM UE
( ) No scars/masses	( ) No JVD	( ) Heme (-) stool	( ) nl ROM LE
( ) nl canals/ TM	( ) nl femoral/pedal	**GU**	L___/5 UE R___/5
( ) nl hearing bilat	pulses	( ) nl ext genitalia	L___/5 LE R___/5
( ) nl teeth/tongue	( ) No pedal	( ) No hernia	
	edema		

+ PE Findings

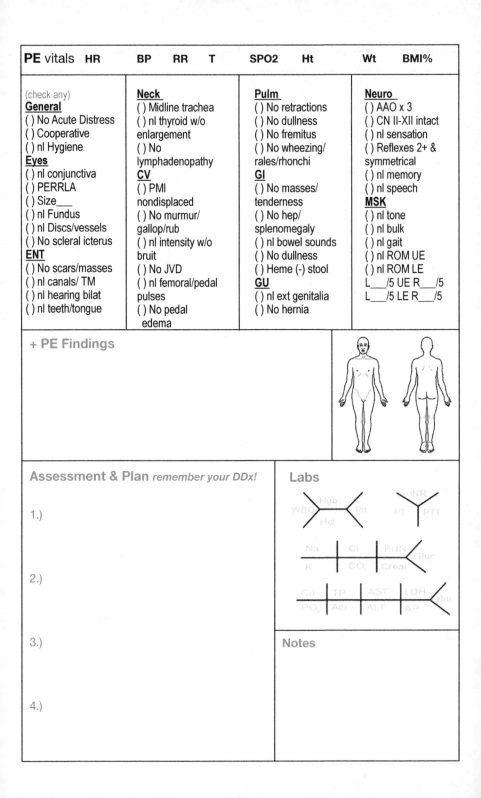

Assessment & Plan *remember your DDx!*

1.)

2.)

3.)

4.)

Labs

Notes

Date: **Initials/MRN:**   **Age:**   **Rotation:**

CC: _____ y/o M/F
HPI: *symptoms/pertinent +/- ROS/prior episodes/recent travel/sick contacts*

PMHx *child/adult illness /hospitalizations/ immunizations*

SurgHx *type/when/ why/complications*

FamHx *parents/siblings/ children*

SHx *smoker/ETOH/illicits/exercise/sex/maritalstatus*

Allergies *meds/foods/ environmental/reactions*

Meds *reason/dose/time/route/compliance/vitamins/ herbs/otcs*

ROS (circle any)

Gen
Fatigue
Weight +/-
Chills
Night sweats
Eyes
Pain
Redness
Vision changes
ENT
Headache
Hoarseness
Sore throat
Sinus sx
Hearing loss
Tinnitus
Runny nose

Pulm
Cough
SOB
Wheezing
Hemoptysis
CV
Chest pain
Edema
PND
Orthopnea
Palpitations
Claudication
GI
Abd pain
N/V
Heartburn
Bloody stools

GU
Dysuria
Frequency
Hematuria
Discharge
Flank pain
MS
Arthralgia
Arthritis
Joint swelling
Myalgias
Back pain
Heme
Bleeding
Bruising
Lymph
Swelling

Endo
Polyuria
Polydypsia
Polyphagia
Derm
Rash
Pruritis
Wound(s)
Neuro
Weakness
Seizures
Parasthesias
Tremors
Syncope
Psych
Anxiety
Depression

+ ROS Findings

PE vitals	**HR**	**BP**	**RR**	**T**	**SPO2**	**Ht**	**Wt**	**BMI%**

(check any)

General
( ) No Acute Distress
( ) Cooperative
( ) nl Hygiene
Eyes
( ) nl conjunctiva
( ) PERRLA
( ) Size___
( ) nl Fundus
( ) nl Discs/vessels
( ) No scleral icterus
ENT
( ) No scars/masses
( ) nl canals/ TM
( ) nl hearing bilat
( ) nl teeth/tongue

Neck
( ) Midline trachea
( ) nl thyroid w/o
enlargement
( ) No
lymphadenopathy
CV
( ) PMI
nondisplaced
( ) No murmur/
gallop/rub
( ) nl intensity w/o
bruit
( ) No JVD
( ) nl femoral/pedal
pulses
( ) No pedal
edema

Pulm
( ) No retractions
( ) No dullness
( ) No fremitus
( ) No wheezing/
rales/rhonchi
GI
( ) No masses/
tenderness
( ) No hep/
splenomegaly
( ) nl bowel sounds
( ) No dullness
( ) Heme (-) stool
GU
( ) nl ext genitalia
( ) No hernia

Neuro
( ) AAO x 3
( ) CN II-XII intact
( ) nl sensation
( ) Reflexes 2+ &
symmetrical
( ) nl memory
( ) nl speech
MSK
( ) nl tone
( ) nl bulk
( ) nl gait
( ) nl ROM UE
( ) nl ROM LE
L___/5 UE R___/5
L___/5 LE R___/5

+ PE Findings

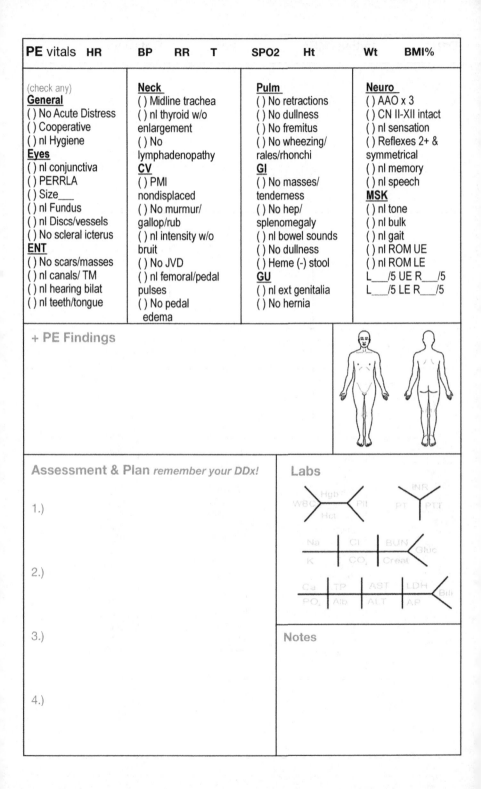

Assessment & Plan *remember your DDx!*

1.)

2.)

3.)

4.)

Labs

Notes

Date:	Initials/MRN:	Age:	Rotation:

CC: _____ y/o M/F
HPI: *symptoms/pertinent +/- ROS/prior episodes/recent travel/sick contacts*

PMHx *child/adult illness /hospitalizations/ immunizations*

SurgHx *type/when/ why/complications*

FamHx *parents/siblings/ children*

SHx *smoker/ETOH/illicits/exercise/sex/maritalstatus*

Allergies *meds/foods/ environmental/reactions*

Meds *reason/dose/time/route/compliance/vitamins/ herbs/otcs*

ROS (circle any)

Gen
Fatigue
Weight +/-
Chills
Night sweats
Eyes
Pain
Redness
Vision changes
ENT
Headache
Hoarseness
Sore throat
Sinus sx
Hearing loss
Tinnitus
Runny nose

Pulm
Cough
SOB
Wheezing
Hemoptysis
CV
Chest pain
Edema
PND
Orthopnea
Palpitations
Claudication
GI
Abd pain
N/V
Heartburn
Bloody stools

GU
Dysuria
Frequency
Hematuria
Discharge
Flank pain
MS
Arthralgia
Arthritis
Joint swelling
Myalgias
Back pain
Heme
Bleeding
Bruising
Lymph
Swelling

Endo
Polyuria
Polydypsia
Polyphagia
Derm
Rash
Pruritis
Wound(s)
Neuro
Weakness
Seizures
Parasthesias
Tremors
Syncope
Psych
Anxiety
Depression

+ ROS Findings

PE vitals **HR**	**BP**	**RR**	**T**	**SPO2**	**Ht**	**Wt**	**BMI%**

(check any) **General** ( ) No Acute Distress ( ) Cooperative ( ) nl Hygiene **Eyes** ( ) nl conjunctiva ( ) PERRLA ( ) Size___ ( ) nl Fundus ( ) nl Discs/vessels ( ) No scleral icterus **ENT** ( ) No scars/masses ( ) nl canals/ TM ( ) nl hearing bilat ( ) nl teeth/tongue	**Neck** ( ) Midline trachea ( ) nl thyroid w/o enlargement ( ) No lymphadenopathy **CV** ( ) PMI nondisplaced ( ) No murmur/ gallop/rub ( ) nl intensity w/o bruit ( ) No JVD ( ) nl femoral/pedal pulses ( ) No pedal edema	**Pulm** ( ) No retractions ( ) No dullness ( ) No fremitus ( ) No wheezing/ rales/rhonchi **GI** ( ) No masses/ tenderness ( ) No hep/ splenomegaly ( ) nl bowel sounds ( ) No dullness ( ) Heme (-) stool **GU** ( ) nl ext genitalia ( ) No hernia	**Neuro** ( ) AAO x 3 ( ) CN II-XII intact ( ) nl sensation ( ) Reflexes 2+ & symmetrical ( ) nl memory ( ) nl speech **MSK** ( ) nl tone ( ) nl bulk ( ) nl gait ( ) nl ROM UE ( ) nl ROM LE L___/5 UE R___/5 L___/5 LE R___/5

+ PE Findings

Assessment & Plan *remember your DDx!*

1.)

2.)

3.)

4.)

Labs

Notes

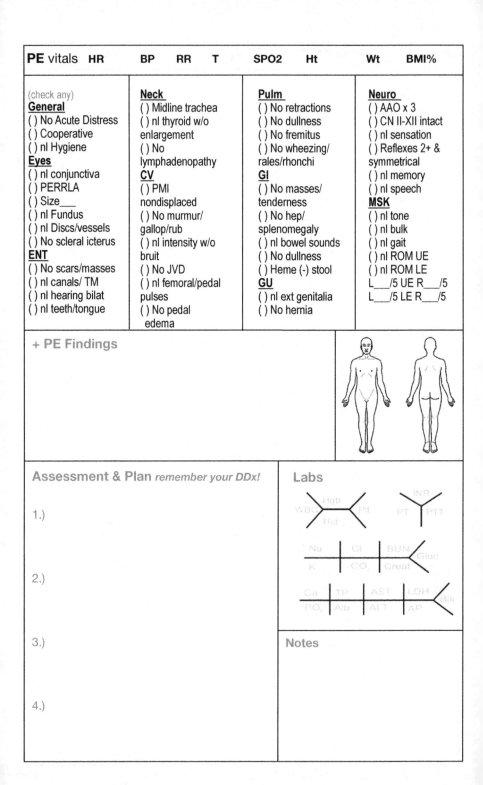

Date:	Initials/MRN:	Age:	Rotation:

CC: _____ y/o M/F
HPI: *symptoms/pertinent +/- ROS/prior episodes/recent travel/sick contacts*

PMHx *child/adult illness /hospitalizations/ immunizations*

SurgHx *type/when/ why/complications*

FamHx *parents/siblings/ children*

SHx *smoker/ETOH/illicits/exercise/sex/maritalstatus*

Allergies *meds/foods/ environmental/reactions*

Meds *reason/dose/time/route/compliance/vitamins/ herbs/otcs*

ROS (circle any)

Gen
Fatigue
Weight +/-
Chills
Night sweats
Eyes
Pain
Redness
Vision changes
ENT
Headache
Hoarseness
Sore throat
Sinus sx
Hearing loss
Tinnitus
Runny nose

Pulm
Cough
SOB
Wheezing
Hemoptysis
CV
Chest pain
Edema
PND
Orthopnea
Palpitations
Claudication
GI
Abd pain
N/V
Heartburn
Bloody stools

GU
Dysuria
Frequency
Hematuria
Discharge
Flank pain
MS
Arthralgia
Arthritis
Joint swelling
Myalgias
Back pain
Heme
Bleeding
Bruising
Lymph
Swelling

Endo
Polyuria
Polydypsia
Polyphagia
Derm
Rash
Pruritis
Wound(s)
Neuro
Weakness
Seizures
Parasthesias
Tremors
Syncope
Psych
Anxiety
Depression

+ ROS Findings

PE vitals **HR**   **BP**   **RR**   **T**   **SPO2**   **Ht**   **Wt**   **BMI%**

(check any)	**Neck**	**Pulm**	**Neuro**
General	( ) Midline trachea	( ) No retractions	( ) AAO x 3
( ) No Acute Distress	( ) nl thyroid w/o	( ) No dullness	( ) CN II-XII intact
( ) Cooperative	enlargement	( ) No fremitus	( ) nl sensation
( ) nl Hygiene	( ) No	( ) No wheezing/	( ) Reflexes 2+ &
Eyes	lymphadenopathy	rales/rhonchi	symmetrical
( ) nl conjunctiva	**CV**	**GI**	( ) nl memory
( ) PERRLA	( ) PMI	( ) No masses/	( ) nl speech
( ) Size___	nondisplaced	tenderness	**MSK**
( ) nl Fundus	( ) No murmur/	( ) No hep/	( ) nl tone
( ) nl Discs/vessels	gallop/rub	splenomegaly	( ) nl bulk
( ) No scleral icterus	( ) nl intensity w/o	( ) nl bowel sounds	( ) nl gait
ENT	bruit	( ) No dullness	( ) nl ROM UE
( ) No scars/masses	( ) No JVD	( ) Heme (-) stool	( ) nl ROM LE
( ) nl canals/ TM	( ) nl femoral/pedal	**GU**	L___/5 UE R___/5
( ) nl hearing bilat	pulses	( ) nl ext genitalia	L___/5 LE R___/5
( ) nl teeth/tongue	( ) No pedal	( ) No hernia	
	edema		

+ PE Findings

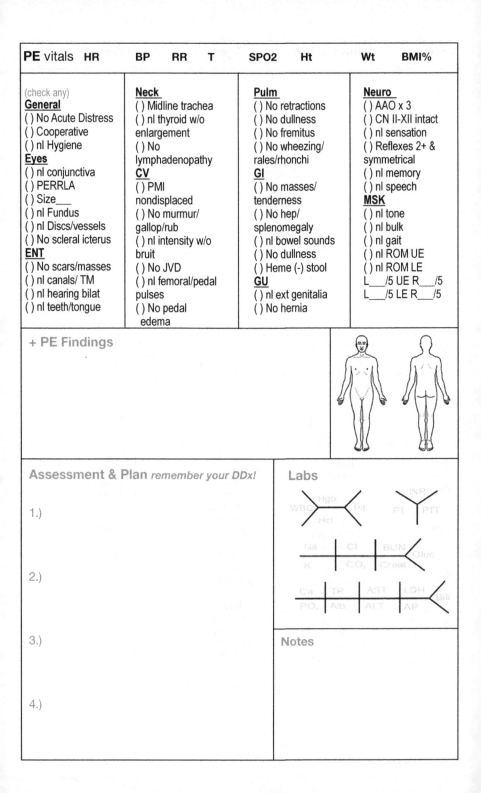

Assessment & Plan *remember your DDx!*

1.)

2.)

3.)

4.)

Labs

Notes

Date:	Initials/MRN:	Age:	Rotation:

CC: _____ y/o M/F

HPI: *symptoms/pertinent +/- ROS/prior episodes/recent travel/sick contacts*

PMHx *child/adult illness /hospitalizations/ immunizations*	**SurgHx** *type/when/ why/complications*	**FamHx** *parents/siblings/ children*

SHx *smoker/ETOH/illicits/exercise/sex/maritalstatus*

Allergies *meds/foods/ environmental/reactions*	**Meds** *reason/dose/time/route/compliance/vitamins/ herbs/otcs*

ROS (circle any)

Gen	**Pulm**	**GU**	**Endo**
Fatigue	Cough	Dysuria	Polyuria
Weight +/-	SOB	Frequency	Polydypsia
Chills	Wheezing	Hematuria	Polyphagia
Night sweats	Hemoptysis	Discharge	**Derm**
Eyes	**CV**	Flank pain	Rash
Pain	Chest pain	**MS**	Pruritis
Redness	Edema	Arthralgia	Wound(s)
Vision changes	PND	Arthritis	**Neuro**
ENT	Orthopnea	Joint swelling	Weakness
Headache	Palpitations	Myalgias	Seizures
Hoarseness	Claudication	Back pain	Parasthesias
Sore throat	**GI**	**Heme**	Tremors
Sinus sx	Abd pain	Bleeding	Syncope
Hearing loss	N/V	Bruising	**Psych**
Tinnitus	Heartburn	**Lymph**	Anxiety
Runny nose	Bloody stools	Swelling	Depression

+ ROS Findings

PE vitals	**HR**	**BP**	**RR**	**T**	**SPO2**	**Ht**	**Wt**	**BMI%**

(check any)

General
( ) No Acute Distress
( ) Cooperative
( ) nl Hygiene
Eyes
( ) nl conjunctiva
( ) PERRLA
( ) Size___
( ) nl Fundus
( ) nl Discs/vessels
( ) No scleral icterus
ENT
( ) No scars/masses
( ) nl canals/ TM
( ) nl hearing bilat
( ) nl teeth/tongue

Neck
( ) Midline trachea
( ) nl thyroid w/o
enlargement
( ) No
lymphadenopathy
CV
( ) PMI
nondisplaced
( ) No murmur/
gallop/rub
( ) nl intensity w/o
bruit
( ) No JVD
( ) nl femoral/pedal
pulses
( ) No pedal
edema

Pulm
( ) No retractions
( ) No dullness
( ) No fremitus
( ) No wheezing/
rales/rhonchi
GI
( ) No masses/
tenderness
( ) No hep/
splenomegaly
( ) nl bowel sounds
( ) No dullness
( ) Heme (-) stool
GU
( ) nl ext genitalia
( ) No hernia

Neuro
( ) AAO x 3
( ) CN II-XII intact
( ) nl sensation
( ) Reflexes 2+ &
symmetrical
( ) nl memory
( ) nl speech
MSK
( ) nl tone
( ) nl bulk
( ) nl gait
( ) nl ROM UE
( ) nl ROM LE
L___/5 UE R___/5
L___/5 LE R___/5

+ PE Findings

Assessment & Plan *remember your DDx!*

1.)

2.)

3.)

4.)

Labs

Notes

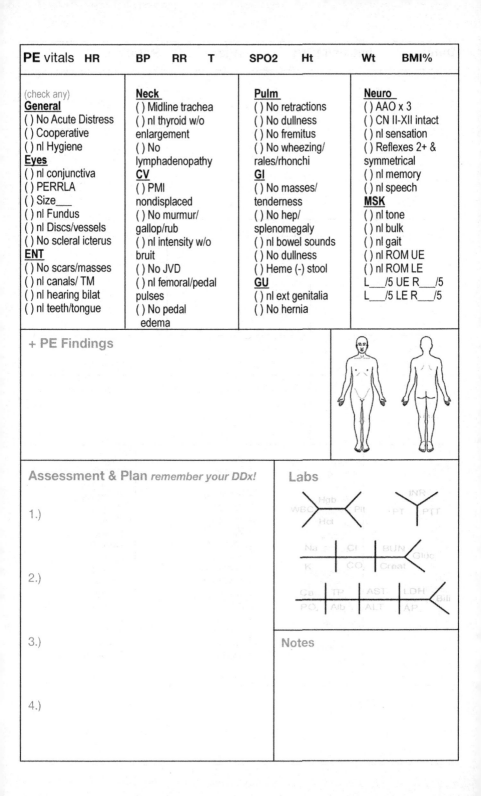

Date: **Initials/MRN:**   **Age:**   **Rotation:**

CC: _____ y/o M/F
HPI: *symptoms/pertinent +/- ROS/prior episodes/recent travel/sick contacts*

PMHx *child/adult illness /hospitalizations/ immunizations*

SurgHx *type/when/ why/complications*

FamHx *parents/siblings/ children*

SHx *smoker/ETOH/illicits/exercise/sex/maritalstatus*

Allergies *meds/foods/ environmental/reactions*

Meds *reason/dose/time/route/compliance/vitamins/ herbs/otcs*

ROS (circle any)

Gen
Fatigue
Weight +/-
Chills
Night sweats
Eyes
Pain
Redness
Vision changes
ENT
Headache
Hoarseness
Sore throat
Sinus sx
Hearing loss
Tinnitus
Runny nose

Pulm
Cough
SOB
Wheezing
Hemoptysis
CV
Chest pain
Edema
PND
Orthopnea
Palpitations
Claudication
GI
Abd pain
N/V
Heartburn
Bloody stools

GU
Dysuria
Frequency
Hematuria
Discharge
Flank pain
MS
Arthralgia
Arthritis
Joint swelling
Myalgias
Back pain
Heme
Bleeding
Bruising
Lymph
Swelling

Endo
Polyuria
Polydypsia
Polyphagia
Derm
Rash
Pruritis
Wound(s)
Neuro
Weakness
Seizures
Parasthesias
Tremors
Syncope
Psych
Anxiety
Depression

+ ROS Findings

PE vitals	**HR**	**BP**	**RR**	**T**	**SPO2**	**Ht**	**Wt**	**BMI%**

(check any)	**Neck**	**Pulm**	**Neuro**
General	( ) Midline trachea	( ) No retractions	( ) AAO x 3
( ) No Acute Distress	( ) nl thyroid w/o	( ) No dullness	( ) CN II-XII intact
( ) Cooperative	enlargement	( ) No fremitus	( ) nl sensation
( ) nl Hygiene	( ) No	( ) No wheezing/	( ) Reflexes 2+ &
Eyes	lymphadenopathy	rales/rhonchi	symmetrical
( ) nl conjunctiva	**CV**	**GI**	( ) nl memory
( ) PERRLA	( ) PMI	( ) No masses/	( ) nl speech
( ) Size___	nondisplaced	tenderness	**MSK**
( ) nl Fundus	( ) No murmur/	( ) No hep/	( ) nl tone
( ) nl Discs/vessels	gallop/rub	splenomegaly	( ) nl bulk
( ) No scleral icterus	( ) nl intensity w/o	( ) nl bowel sounds	( ) nl gait
ENT	bruit	( ) No dullness	( ) nl ROM UE
( ) No scars/masses	( ) No JVD	( ) Heme (-) stool	( ) nl ROM LE
( ) nl canals/ TM	( ) nl femoral/pedal	**GU**	L___/5 UE R___/5
( ) nl hearing bilat	pulses	( ) nl ext genitalia	L___/5 LE R___/5
( ) nl teeth/tongue	( ) No pedal	( ) No hernia	
	edema		

+ PE Findings

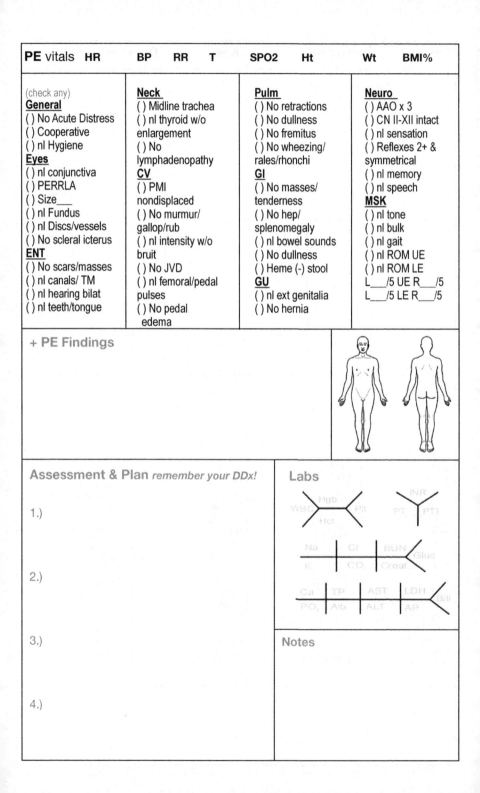

Assessment & Plan *remember your DDx!*

1.)

2.)

3.)

4.)

Labs

Notes

Date:	Initials/MRN:	Age:	Rotation:

CC: _____ y/o M/F
HPI: *symptoms/pertinent +/- ROS/prior episodes/recent travel/sick contacts*

PMHx *child/adult illness /hospitalizations/ immunizations*

SurgHx *type/when/ why/complications*

FamHx *parents/siblings/ children*

SHx *smoker/ETOH/illicits/exercise/sex/maritalstatus*

Allergies *meds/foods/ environmental/reactions*

Meds *reason/dose/time/route/compliance/vitamins/ herbs/otcs*

ROS (circle any)

Gen
Fatigue
Weight +/-
Chills
Night sweats
Eyes
Pain
Redness
Vision changes
ENT
Headache
Hoarseness
Sore throat
Sinus sx
Hearing loss
Tinnitus
Runny nose

Pulm
Cough
SOB
Wheezing
Hemoptysis
CV
Chest pain
Edema
PND
Orthopnea
Palpitations
Claudication
GI
Abd pain
N/V
Heartburn
Bloody stools

GU
Dysuria
Frequency
Hematuria
Discharge
Flank pain
MS
Arthralgia
Arthritis
Joint swelling
Myalgias
Back pain
Heme
Bleeding
Bruising
Lymph
Swelling

Endo
Polyuria
Polydypsia
Polyphagia
Derm
Rash
Pruritis
Wound(s)
Neuro
Weakness
Seizures
Parasthesias
Tremors
Syncope
Psych
Anxiety
Depression

+ ROS Findings

PE vitals	HR	BP	RR	T	SPO2	Ht	Wt	BMI%

(check any)

General
( ) No Acute Distress
( ) Cooperative
( ) nl Hygiene
Eyes
( ) nl conjunctiva
( ) PERRLA
( ) Size___
( ) nl Fundus
( ) nl Discs/vessels
( ) No scleral icterus
ENT
( ) No scars/masses
( ) nl canals/ TM
( ) nl hearing bilat
( ) nl teeth/tongue

Neck
( ) Midline trachea
( ) nl thyroid w/o enlargement
( ) No lymphadenopathy
CV
( ) PMI nondisplaced
( ) No murmur/ gallop/rub
( ) nl intensity w/o bruit
( ) No JVD
( ) nl femoral/pedal pulses
( ) No pedal edema

Pulm
( ) No retractions
( ) No dullness
( ) No fremitus
( ) No wheezing/ rales/rhonchi
GI
( ) No masses/ tenderness
( ) No hep/ splenomegaly
( ) nl bowel sounds
( ) No dullness
( ) Heme (-) stool
GU
( ) nl ext genitalia
( ) No hernia

Neuro
( ) AAO x 3
( ) CN II-XII intact
( ) nl sensation
( ) Reflexes 2+ & symmetrical
( ) nl memory
( ) nl speech
MSK
( ) nl tone
( ) nl bulk
( ) nl gait
( ) nl ROM UE
( ) nl ROM LE
L___/5 UE R___/5
L___/5 LE R___/5

+ PE Findings

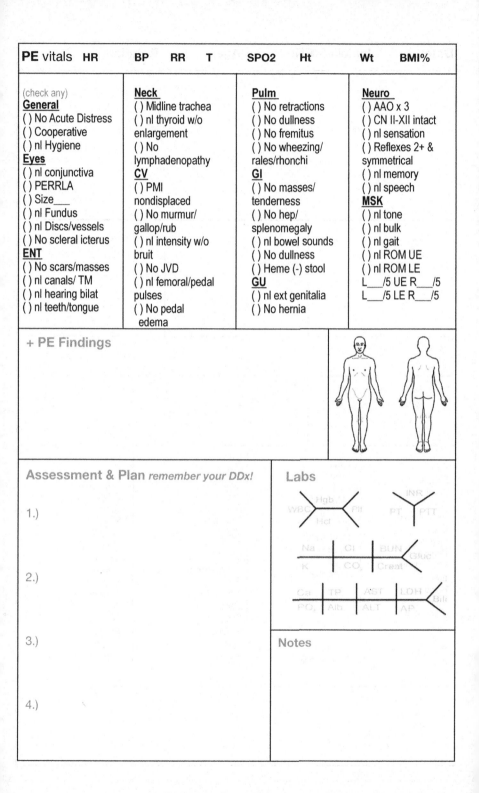

Assessment & Plan *remember your DDx!*

1.)

2.)

3.)

4.)

Labs

Notes

Date: **Initials/MRN:**   **Age:**   **Rotation:**

CC: _____ y/o M/F
HPI: *symptoms/pertinent +/- ROS/prior episodes/recent travel/sick contacts*

PMHx *child/adult illness /hospitalizations/ immunizations*	**SurgHx** *type/when/ why/complications*	**FamHx** *parents/siblings/ children*

SHx *smoker/ETOH/illicits/exercise/sex/maritalstatus*

Allergies *meds/foods/ environmental/reactions*	**Meds** *reason/dose/time/route/compliance/vitamins/ herbs/otcs*

ROS (circle any)

Gen	**Pulm**	**GU**	**Endo**
Fatigue	Cough	Dysuria	Polyuria
Weight +/-	SOB	Frequency	Polydypsia
Chills	Wheezing	Hematuria	Polyphagia
Night sweats	Hemoptysis	Discharge	**Derm**
Eyes	**CV**	Flank pain	Rash
Pain	Chest pain	**MS**	Pruritis
Redness	Edema	Arthralgia	Wound(s)
Vision changes	PND	Arthritis	**Neuro**
ENT	Orthopnea	Joint swelling	Weakness
Headache	Palpitations	Myalgias	Seizures
Hoarseness	Claudication	Back pain	Parasthesias
Sore throat	**GI**	**Heme**	Tremors
Sinus sx	Abd pain	Bleeding	Syncope
Hearing loss	N/V	Bruising	**Psych**
Tinnitus	Heartburn	**Lymph**	Anxiety
Runny nose	Bloody stools	Swelling	Depression

+ ROS Findings

PE vitals	HR	BP	RR	T	SPO2	Ht	Wt	BMI%

(check any)

General
( ) No Acute Distress
( ) Cooperative
( ) nl Hygiene
Eyes
( ) nl conjunctiva
( ) PERRLA
( ) Size___
( ) nl Fundus
( ) nl Discs/vessels
( ) No scleral icterus
ENT
( ) No scars/masses
( ) nl canals/ TM
( ) nl hearing bilat
( ) nl teeth/tongue

Neck
( ) Midline trachea
( ) nl thyroid w/o enlargement
( ) No lymphadenopathy
CV
( ) PMI nondisplaced
( ) No murmur/ gallop/rub
( ) nl intensity w/o bruit
( ) No JVD
( ) nl femoral/pedal pulses
( ) No pedal edema

Pulm
( ) No retractions
( ) No dullness
( ) No fremitus
( ) No wheezing/ rales/rhonchi
GI
( ) No masses/ tenderness
( ) No hep/ splenomegaly
( ) nl bowel sounds
( ) No dullness
( ) Heme (-) stool
GU
( ) nl ext genitalia
( ) No hernia

Neuro
( ) AAO x 3
( ) CN II-XII intact
( ) nl sensation
( ) Reflexes 2+ & symmetrical
( ) nl memory
( ) nl speech
MSK
( ) nl tone
( ) nl bulk
( ) nl gait
( ) nl ROM UE
( ) nl ROM LE
L___/5 UE R___/5
L___/5 LE R___/5

+ PE Findings

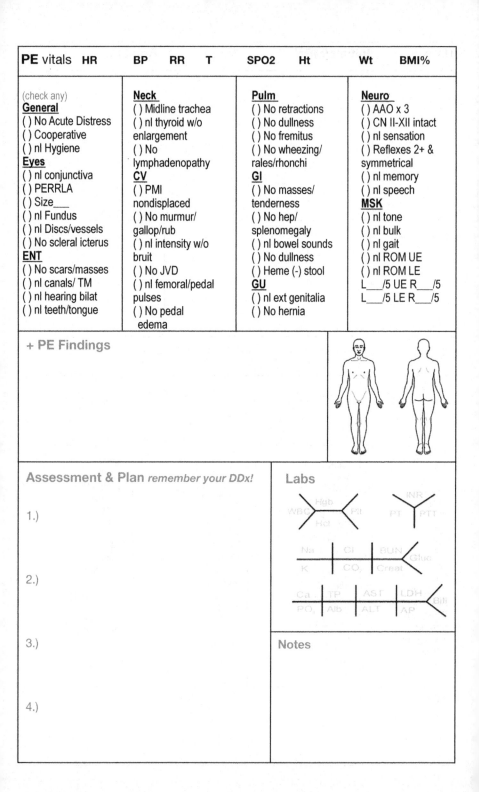

Assessment & Plan *remember your DDx!*

1.)

2.)

3.)

4.)

Labs

Hgb
WBC   Plt
Hct

INR
PT   PTT

Na   Cl   BUN
        Gluc
K   CO₂   Creat

Ca   TP   AST   LDH
            Bili
PO₄   Alb   ALT   AP

Notes

Date:	Initials/MRN:	Age:	Rotation:

CC: _____ y/o M/F
HPI: *symptoms/pertinent +/- ROS/prior episodes/recent travel/sick contacts*

PMHx *child/adult illness /hospitalizations/ immunizations*	**SurgHx** *type/when/ why/complications*	**FamHx** *parents/siblings/ children*

SHx *smoker/ETOH/illicits/exercise/sex/maritalstatus*

Allergies *meds/foods/ environmental/reactions*	**Meds** *reason/dose/time/route/compliance/vitamins/ herbs/otcs*

ROS (circle any)

Gen	**Pulm**	**GU**	**Endo**
Fatigue	Cough	Dysuria	Polyuria
Weight +/-	SOB	Frequency	Polydypsia
Chills	Wheezing	Hematuria	Polyphagia
Night sweats	Hemoptysis	Discharge	**Derm**
Eyes	**CV**	Flank pain	Rash
Pain	Chest pain	**MS**	Pruritis
Redness	Edema	Arthralgia	Wound(s)
Vision changes	PND	Arthritis	**Neuro**
ENT	Orthopnea	Joint swelling	Weakness
Headache	Palpitations	Myalgias	Seizures
Hoarseness	Claudication	Back pain	Parasthesias
Sore throat	**GI**	**Heme**	Tremors
Sinus sx	Abd pain	Bleeding	Syncope
Hearing loss	N/V	Bruising	**Psych**
Tinnitus	Heartburn	**Lymph**	Anxiety
Runny nose	Bloody stools	Swelling	Depression

+ ROS Findings

PE vitals	**HR**	**BP**	**RR**	**T**	**SPO2**	**Ht**	**Wt**	**BMI%**

(check any)	**Neck**	**Pulm**	**Neuro**
General	( ) Midline trachea	( ) No retractions	( ) AAO x 3
( ) No Acute Distress	( ) nl thyroid w/o	( ) No dullness	( ) CN II-XII intact
( ) Cooperative	enlargement	( ) No fremitus	( ) nl sensation
( ) nl Hygiene	( ) No	( ) No wheezing/	( ) Reflexes 2+ &
Eyes	lymphadenopathy	rales/rhonchi	symmetrical
( ) nl conjunctiva	**CV**	**GI**	( ) nl memory
( ) PERRLA	( ) PMI	( ) No masses/	( ) nl speech
( ) Size___	nondisplaced	tenderness	**MSK**
( ) nl Fundus	( ) No murmur/	( ) No hep/	( ) nl tone
( ) nl Discs/vessels	gallop/rub	splenomegaly	( ) nl bulk
( ) No scleral icterus	( ) nl intensity w/o	( ) nl bowel sounds	( ) nl gait
ENT	bruit	( ) No dullness	( ) nl ROM UE
( ) No scars/masses	( ) No JVD	( ) Heme (-) stool	( ) nl ROM LE
( ) nl canals/ TM	( ) nl femoral/pedal	**GU**	L___/5 UE R___/5
( ) nl hearing bilat	pulses	( ) nl ext genitalia	L___/5 LE R___/5
( ) nl teeth/tongue	( ) No pedal	( ) No hernia	
	edema		

+ PE Findings

Assessment & Plan *remember your DDx!*

1.)

2.)

3.)

4.)

Labs

Notes

Date:	Initials/MRN:	Age:	Rotation:

CC: _____ y/o M/F
HPI: *symptoms/pertinent +/- ROS/prior episodes/recent travel/sick contacts*

PMHx *child/adult illness /hospitalizations/ immunizations*	**SurgHx** *type/when/ why/complications*	**FamHx** *parents/siblings/ children*

SHx *smoker/ETOH/illicits/exercise/sex/maritalstatus*

Allergies *meds/foods/ environmental/reactions*	**Meds** *reason/dose/time/route/compliance/vitamins/ herbs/otcs*

ROS (circle any)

Gen	**Pulm**	**GU**	**Endo**
Fatigue	Cough	Dysuria	Polyuria
Weight +/-	SOB	Frequency	Polydypsia
Chills	Wheezing	Hematuria	Polyphagia
Night sweats	Hemoptysis	Discharge	**Derm**
Eyes	**CV**	Flank pain	Rash
Pain	Chest pain	**MS**	Pruritis
Redness	Edema	Arthralgia	Wound(s)
Vision changes	PND	Arthritis	**Neuro**
ENT	Orthopnea	Joint swelling	Weakness
Headache	Palpitations	Myalgias	Seizures
Hoarseness	Claudication	Back pain	Parasthesias
Sore throat	**GI**	**Heme**	Tremors
Sinus sx	Abd pain	Bleeding	Syncope
Hearing loss	N/V	Bruising	**Psych**
Tinnitus	Heartburn	**Lymph**	Anxiety
Runny nose	Bloody stools	Swelling	Depression

+ ROS Findings

PE vitals	HR	BP	RR	T	SPO2	Ht	Wt	BMI%

(check any)

General
( ) No Acute Distress
( ) Cooperative
( ) nl Hygiene

Eyes
( ) nl conjunctiva
( ) PERRLA
( ) Size___
( ) nl Fundus
( ) nl Discs/vessels
( ) No scleral icterus

ENT
( ) No scars/masses
( ) nl canals/ TM
( ) nl hearing bilat
( ) nl teeth/tongue

Neck
( ) Midline trachea
( ) nl thyroid w/o
enlargement
( ) No
lymphadenopathy

CV
( ) PMI
nondisplaced
( ) No murmur/
gallop/rub
( ) nl intensity w/o
bruit
( ) No JVD
( ) nl femoral/pedal
pulses
( ) No pedal
edema

Pulm
( ) No retractions
( ) No dullness
( ) No fremitus
( ) No wheezing/
rales/rhonchi

GI
( ) No masses/
tenderness
( ) No hep/
splenomegaly
( ) nl bowel sounds
( ) No dullness
( ) Heme (-) stool

GU
( ) nl ext genitalia
( ) No hernia

Neuro
( ) AAO x 3
( ) CN II-XII intact
( ) nl sensation
( ) Reflexes 2+ &
symmetrical
( ) nl memory
( ) nl speech

MSK
( ) nl tone
( ) nl bulk
( ) nl gait
( ) nl ROM UE
( ) nl ROM LE
L___/5 UE R___/5
L___/5 LE R___/5

+ PE Findings

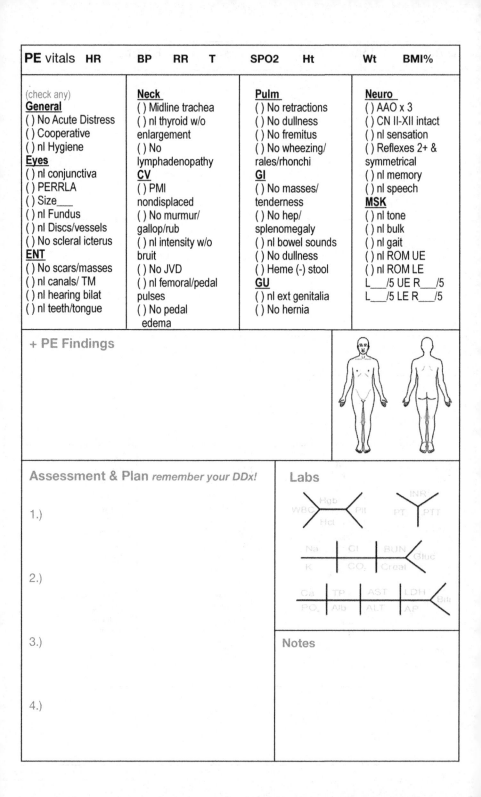

Assessment & Plan *remember your DDx!*

1.)

2.)

3.)

4.)

Labs

Notes

Date:	Initials/MRN:	Age:	Rotation:

CC: _____ y/o M/F
HPI: *symptoms/pertinent +/- ROS/prior episodes/recent travel/sick contacts*

PMHx *child/adult illness /hospitalizations/ immunizations*	**SurgHx** *type/when/ why/complications*	**FamHx** *parents/siblings/ children*

SHx *smoker/ETOH/illicits/exercise/sex/maritalstatus*

Allergies *meds/foods/ environmental/reactions*	**Meds** *reason/dose/time/route/compliance/vitamins/ herbs/otcs*

ROS (circle any)

Gen	**Pulm**	**GU**	**Endo**
Fatigue	Cough	Dysuria	Polyuria
Weight +/-	SOB	Frequency	Polydypsia
Chills	Wheezing	Hematuria	Polyphagia
Night sweats	Hemoptysis	Discharge	**Derm**
Eyes	**CV**	Flank pain	Rash
Pain	Chest pain	**MS**	Pruritis
Redness	Edema	Arthralgia	Wound(s)
Vision changes	PND	Arthritis	**Neuro**
ENT	Orthopnea	Joint swelling	Weakness
Headache	Palpitations	Myalgias	Seizures
Hoarseness	Claudication	Back pain	Parasthesias
Sore throat	**GI**	**Heme**	Tremors
Sinus sx	Abd pain	Bleeding	Syncope
Hearing loss	N/V	Bruising	**Psych**
Tinnitus	Heartburn	**Lymph**	Anxiety
Runny nose	Bloody stools	Swelling	Depression

+ ROS Findings

PE vitals	HR	BP	RR	T	SPO2	Ht	Wt	BMI%

(check any)

General
( ) No Acute Distress
( ) Cooperative
( ) nl Hygiene
Eyes
( ) nl conjunctiva
( ) PERRLA
( ) Size___
( ) nl Fundus
( ) nl Discs/vessels
( ) No scleral icterus
ENT
( ) No scars/masses
( ) nl canals/ TM
( ) nl hearing bilat
( ) nl teeth/tongue

Neck
( ) Midline trachea
( ) nl thyroid w/o
enlargement
( ) No
lymphadenopathy
CV
( ) PMI
nondisplaced
( ) No murmur/
gallop/rub
( ) nl intensity w/o
bruit
( ) No JVD
( ) nl femoral/pedal
pulses
( ) No pedal
edema

Pulm
( ) No retractions
( ) No dullness
( ) No fremitus
( ) No wheezing/
rales/rhonchi
GI
( ) No masses/
tenderness
( ) No hep/
splenomegaly
( ) nl bowel sounds
( ) No dullness
( ) Heme (-) stool
GU
( ) nl ext genitalia
( ) No hernia

Neuro
( ) AAO x 3
( ) CN II-XII intact
( ) nl sensation
( ) Reflexes 2+ &
symmetrical
( ) nl memory
( ) nl speech
MSK
( ) nl tone
( ) nl bulk
( ) nl gait
( ) nl ROM UE
( ) nl ROM LE
L___/5 UE R___/5
L___/5 LE R___/5

+ PE Findings

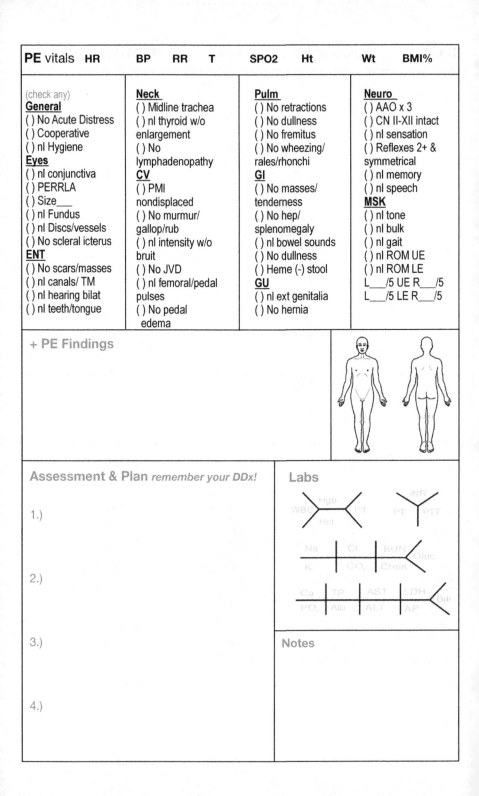

Assessment & Plan *remember your DDx!*

1.)

2.)

3.)

4.)

Labs

Hgb
WBC   Plt
Hct

INR
PT   PTT

Na   Cl   BUN
  Gluc
K   CO₂   Creat

Ca   TP   AST   LDH
  Bili
PO₄   Alb   ALT   AP

Notes

Date:	Initials/MRN:	Age:	Rotation:

CC: _____ y/o M/F
HPI: *symptoms/pertinent +/- ROS/prior episodes/recent travel/sick contacts*

PMHx *child/adult illness /hospitalizations/ immunizations*	**SurgHx** *type/when/ why/complications*	**FamHx** *parents/siblings/ children*

SHx *smoker/ETOH/illicits/exercise/sex/maritalstatus*

Allergies *meds/foods/ environmental/reactions*	**Meds** *reason/dose/time/route/compliance/vitamins/ herbs/otcs*

ROS (circle any)

Gen	**Pulm**	**GU**	**Endo**
Fatigue	Cough	Dysuria	Polyuria
Weight +/-	SOB	Frequency	Polydypsia
Chills	Wheezing	Hematuria	Polyphagia
Night sweats	Hemoptysis	Discharge	**Derm**
Eyes	**CV**	Flank pain	Rash
Pain	Chest pain	**MS**	Pruritis
Redness	Edema	Arthralgia	Wound(s)
Vision changes	PND	Arthritis	**Neuro**
ENT	Orthopnea	Joint swelling	Weakness
Headache	Palpitations	Myalgias	Seizures
Hoarseness	Claudication	Back pain	Parasthesias
Sore throat	**GI**	**Heme**	Tremors
Sinus sx	Abd pain	Bleeding	Syncope
Hearing loss	N/V	Bruising	**Psych**
Tinnitus	Heartburn	**Lymph**	Anxiety
Runny nose	Bloody stools	Swelling	Depression

+ ROS Findings

PE vitals	**HR**	**BP**	**RR**	**T**	**SPO2**	**Ht**	**Wt**	**BMI%**

(check any)

General
( ) No Acute Distress
( ) Cooperative
( ) nl Hygiene
Eyes
( ) nl conjunctiva
( ) PERRLA
( ) Size___
( ) nl Fundus
( ) nl Discs/vessels
( ) No scleral icterus
ENT
( ) No scars/masses
( ) nl canals/ TM
( ) nl hearing bilat
( ) nl teeth/tongue

Neck
( ) Midline trachea
( ) nl thyroid w/o enlargement
( ) No lymphadenopathy
CV
( ) PMI nondisplaced
( ) No murmur/ gallop/rub
( ) nl intensity w/o bruit
( ) No JVD
( ) nl femoral/pedal pulses
( ) No pedal edema

Pulm
( ) No retractions
( ) No dullness
( ) No fremitus
( ) No wheezing/ rales/rhonchi
GI
( ) No masses/ tenderness
( ) No hep/ splenomegaly
( ) nl bowel sounds
( ) No dullness
( ) Heme (-) stool
GU
( ) nl ext genitalia
( ) No hernia

Neuro
( ) AAO x 3
( ) CN II-XII intact
( ) nl sensation
( ) Reflexes 2+ & symmetrical
( ) nl memory
( ) nl speech
MSK
( ) nl tone
( ) nl bulk
( ) nl gait
( ) nl ROM UE
( ) nl ROM LE
L___/5 UE R___/5
L___/5 LE R___/5

+ PE Findings

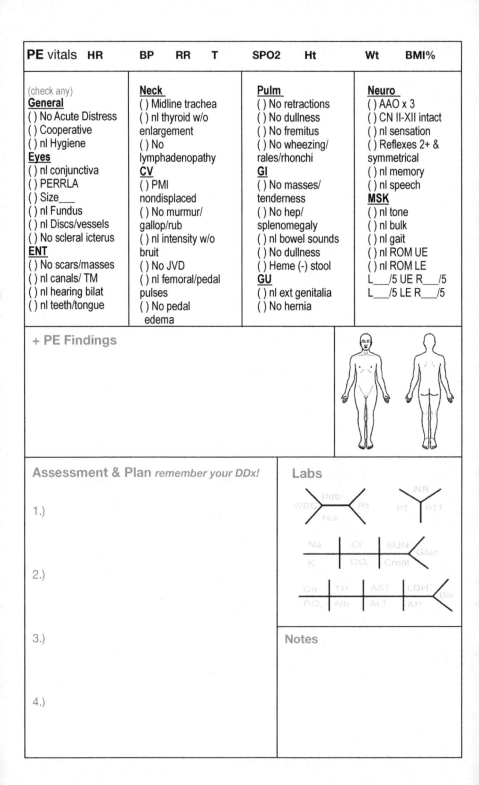

Assessment & Plan *remember your DDx!*

1.)

2.)

3.)

4.)

Labs

Hgb
WBC — Plt
Hct

INR
PT — PTT

Na | Cl | BUN
K | CO2 | Creat — Gluc

Ca | TP | AST | LDH
PO4 | Alb | ALT | AP — Bili

Notes

Date: **Initials/MRN:**   **Age:**   **Rotation:**

CC: _____ y/o M/F
HPI: *symptoms/pertinent +/- ROS/prior episodes/recent travel/sick contacts*

PMHx *child/adult illness /hospitalizations/ immunizations*

SurgHx *type/when/ why/complications*

FamHx *parents/siblings/ children*

SHx *smoker/ETOH/illicits/exercise/sex/maritalstatus*

Allergies *meds/foods/ environmental/reactions*

Meds *reason/dose/time/route/compliance/vitamins/ herbs/otcs*

ROS (circle any)

Gen
Fatigue
Weight +/-
Chills
Night sweats
Eyes
Pain
Redness
Vision changes
ENT
Headache
Hoarseness
Sore throat
Sinus sx
Hearing loss
Tinnitus
Runny nose

Pulm
Cough
SOB
Wheezing
Hemoptysis
CV
Chest pain
Edema
PND
Orthopnea
Palpitations
Claudication
GI
Abd pain
N/V
Heartburn
Bloody stools

GU
Dysuria
Frequency
Hematuria
Discharge
Flank pain
MS
Arthralgia
Arthritis
Joint swelling
Myalgias
Back pain
Heme
Bleeding
Bruising
Lymph
Swelling

Endo
Polyuria
Polydypsia
Polyphagia
Derm
Rash
Pruritis
Wound(s)
Neuro
Weakness
Seizures
Parasthesias
Tremors
Syncope
Psych
Anxiety
Depression

+ ROS Findings

PE vitals	**HR**	**BP**	**RR**	**T**	**SPO2**	**Ht**	**Wt**	**BMI%**

(check any)	**Neck**	**Pulm**	**Neuro**
General	( ) Midline trachea	( ) No retractions	( ) AAO x 3
( ) No Acute Distress	( ) nl thyroid w/o	( ) No dullness	( ) CN II-XII intact
( ) Cooperative	enlargement	( ) No fremitus	( ) nl sensation
( ) nl Hygiene	( ) No	( ) No wheezing/	( ) Reflexes 2+ &
Eyes	lymphadenopathy	rales/rhonchi	symmetrical
( ) nl conjunctiva	**CV**	**GI**	( ) nl memory
( ) PERRLA	( ) PMI	( ) No masses/	( ) nl speech
( ) Size___	nondisplaced	tenderness	**MSK**
( ) nl Fundus	( ) No murmur/	( ) No hep/	( ) nl tone
( ) nl Discs/vessels	gallop/rub	splenomegaly	( ) nl bulk
( ) No scleral icterus	( ) nl intensity w/o	( ) nl bowel sounds	( ) nl gait
ENT	bruit	( ) No dullness	( ) nl ROM UE
( ) No scars/masses	( ) No JVD	( ) Heme (-) stool	( ) nl ROM LE
( ) nl canals/ TM	( ) nl femoral/pedal	**GU**	L___/5 UE R___/5
( ) nl hearing bilat	pulses	( ) nl ext genitalia	L___/5 LE R___/5
( ) nl teeth/tongue	( ) No pedal	( ) No hernia	
	edema		

+ PE Findings

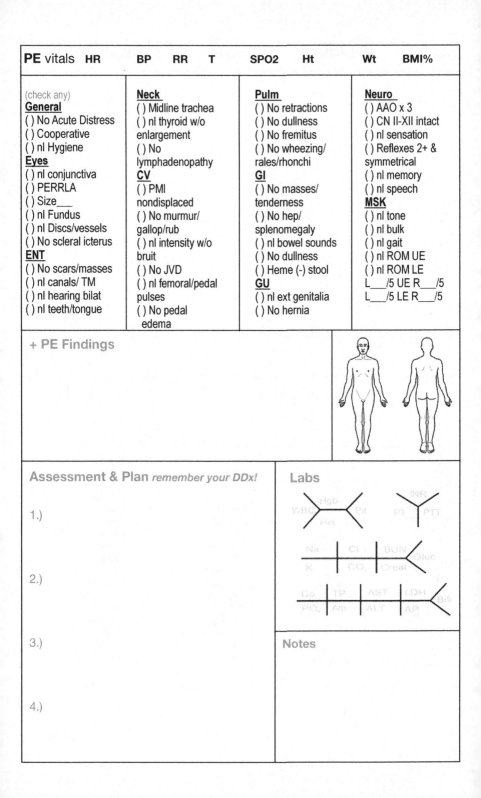

Assessment & Plan *remember your DDx!*

1.)

2.)

3.)

4.)

Labs

Notes

Date: **Initials/MRN:**   **Age:**   **Rotation:**

CC: _____ y/o M/F
HPI: *symptoms/pertinent +/- ROS/prior episodes/recent travel/sick contacts*

PMHx *child/adult illness /hospitalizations/ immunizations*

SurgHx *type/when/ why/complications*

FamHx *parents/siblings/ children*

SHx *smoker/ETOH/illicits/exercise/sex/maritalstatus*

Allergies *meds/foods/ environmental/reactions*

Meds *reason/dose/time/route/compliance/vitamins/ herbs/otcs*

ROS (circle any)

Gen	Pulm	GU	Endo
Fatigue	Cough	Dysuria	Polyuria
Weight +/-	SOB	Frequency	Polydypsia
Chills	Wheezing	Hematuria	Polyphagia
Night sweats	Hemoptysis	Discharge	**Derm**
Eyes	**CV**	Flank pain	Rash
Pain	Chest pain	**MS**	Pruritis
Redness	Edema	Arthralgia	Wound(s)
Vision changes	PND	Arthritis	**Neuro**
ENT	Orthopnea	Joint swelling	Weakness
Headache	Palpitations	Myalgias	Seizures
Hoarseness	Claudication	Back pain	Parasthesias
Sore throat	**GI**	**Heme**	Tremors
Sinus sx	Abd pain	Bleeding	Syncope
Hearing loss	N/V	Bruising	**Psych**
Tinnitus	Heartburn	**Lymph**	Anxiety
Runny nose	Bloody stools	Swelling	Depression

+ ROS Findings

PE vitals HR	BP	RR	T	SPO2	Ht	Wt	BMI%

(check any)	**Neck**	**Pulm**	**Neuro**
General	( ) Midline trachea	( ) No retractions	( ) AAO x 3
( ) No Acute Distress	( ) nl thyroid w/o	( ) No dullness	( ) CN II-XII intact
( ) Cooperative	enlargement	( ) No fremitus	( ) nl sensation
( ) nl Hygiene	( ) No	( ) No wheezing/	( ) Reflexes 2+ &
Eyes	lymphadenopathy	rales/rhonchi	symmetrical
( ) nl conjunctiva	**CV**	**GI**	( ) nl memory
( ) PERRLA	( ) PMI	( ) No masses/	( ) nl speech
( ) Size___	nondisplaced	tenderness	**MSK**
( ) nl Fundus	( ) No murmur/	( ) No hep/	( ) nl tone
( ) nl Discs/vessels	gallop/rub	splenomegaly	( ) nl bulk
( ) No scleral icterus	( ) nl intensity w/o	( ) nl bowel sounds	( ) nl gait
ENT	bruit	( ) No dullness	( ) nl ROM UE
( ) No scars/masses	( ) No JVD	( ) Heme (-) stool	( ) nl ROM LE
( ) nl canals/ TM	( ) nl femoral/pedal	**GU**	L___/5 UE R___/5
( ) nl hearing bilat	pulses	( ) nl ext genitalia	L___/5 LE R___/5
( ) nl teeth/tongue	( ) No pedal	( ) No hernia	
	edema		

+ PE Findings

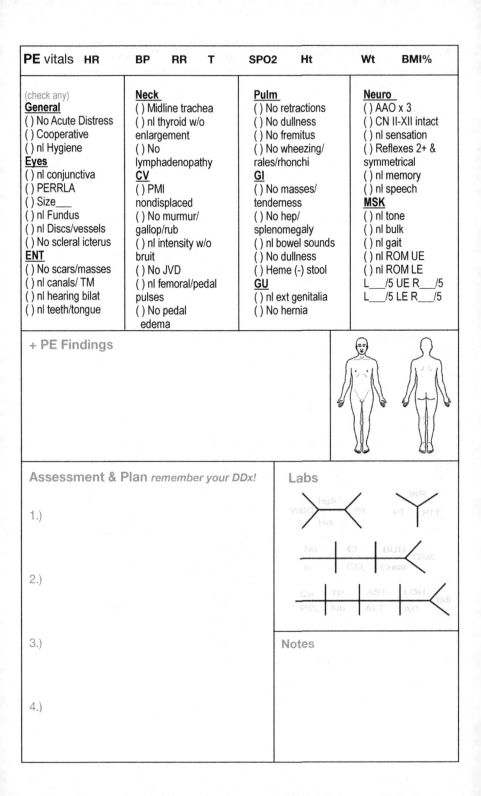

Assessment & Plan *remember your DDx!*

1.)

2.)

3.)

4.)

Labs

Notes

Date:	Initials/MRN:	Age:	Rotation:

CC: _____ y/o M/F
HPI: *symptoms/pertinent +/- ROS/prior episodes/recent travel/sick contacts*

PMHx *child/adult illness /hospitalizations/ immunizations*

SurgHx *type/when/ why/complications*

FamHx *parents/siblings/ children*

SHx *smoker/ETOH/illicits/exercise/sex/maritalstatus*

Allergies *meds/foods/ environmental/reactions*

Meds *reason/dose/time/route/compliance/vitamins/ herbs/otcs*

ROS (circle any)

Gen
Fatigue
Weight +/-
Chills
Night sweats
Eyes
Pain
Redness
Vision changes
ENT
Headache
Hoarseness
Sore throat
Sinus sx
Hearing loss
Tinnitus
Runny nose

Pulm
Cough
 SOB
 Wheezing
 Hemoptysis
CV
Chest pain
 Edema
 PND
 Orthopnea
 Palpitations
 Claudication
GI
Abd pain
N/V
Heartburn
Bloody stools

GU
Dysuria
Frequency
Hematuria
Discharge
Flank pain
MS
 Arthralgia
 Arthritis
 Joint swelling
 Myalgias
 Back pain
Heme
Bleeding
Bruising
Lymph
Swelling

Endo
Polyuria
Polydypsia
Polyphagia
Derm
Rash
Pruritis
Wound(s)
Neuro
Weakness
Seizures
Parasthesias
Tremors
Syncope
Psych
Anxiety
Depression

+ ROS Findings

PE vitals	HR	BP	RR	T	SPO2	Ht	Wt	BMI%

(check any)

General
( ) No Acute Distress
( ) Cooperative
( ) nl Hygiene
Eyes
( ) nl conjunctiva
( ) PERRLA
( ) Size___
( ) nl Fundus
( ) nl Discs/vessels
( ) No scleral icterus
ENT
( ) No scars/masses
( ) nl canals/ TM
( ) nl hearing bilat
( ) nl teeth/tongue

Neck
( ) Midline trachea
( ) nl thyroid w/o enlargement
( ) No lymphadenopathy
CV
( ) PMI nondisplaced
( ) No murmur/ gallop/rub
( ) nl intensity w/o bruit
( ) No JVD
( ) nl femoral/pedal pulses
( ) No pedal edema

Pulm
( ) No retractions
( ) No dullness
( ) No fremitus
( ) No wheezing/ rales/rhonchi
GI
( ) No masses/ tenderness
( ) No hep/ splenomegaly
( ) nl bowel sounds
( ) No dullness
( ) Heme (-) stool
GU
( ) nl ext genitalia
( ) No hernia

Neuro
( ) AAO x 3
( ) CN II-XII intact
( ) nl sensation
( ) Reflexes 2+ & symmetrical
( ) nl memory
( ) nl speech
MSK
( ) nl tone
( ) nl bulk
( ) nl gait
( ) nl ROM UE
( ) nl ROM LE
L___/5 UE R___/5
L___/5 LE R___/5

+ PE Findings

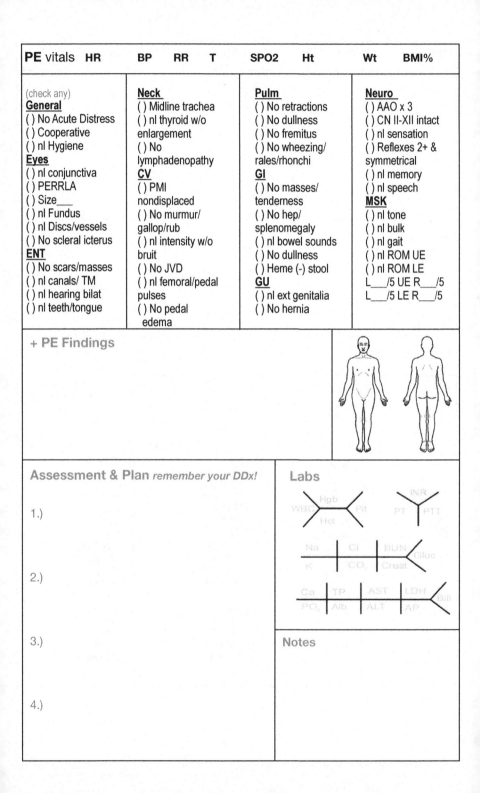

Assessment & Plan *remember your DDx!*

1.)

2.)

3.)

4.)

Labs

Notes

Date:	Initials/MRN:	Age:	Rotation:

CC: _____ y/o M/F
HPI: *symptoms/pertinent +/- ROS/prior episodes/recent travel/sick contacts*

PMHx *child/adult illness /hospitalizations/ immunizations*

SurgHx *type/when/ why/complications*

FamHx *parents/siblings/ children*

SHx *smoker/ETOH/illicits/exercise/sex/maritalstatus*

Allergies *meds/foods/ environmental/reactions*

Meds *reason/dose/time/route/compliance/vitamins/ herbs/otcs*

ROS (circle any)

Gen
Fatigue
Weight +/-
Chills
Night sweats
Eyes
Pain
Redness
Vision changes
ENT
Headache
Hoarseness
Sore throat
Sinus sx
Hearing loss
Tinnitus
Runny nose

Pulm
Cough
SOB
Wheezing
Hemoptysis
CV
Chest pain
Edema
PND
Orthopnea
Palpitations
Claudication
GI
Abd pain
N/V
Heartburn
Bloody stools

GU
Dysuria
Frequency
Hematuria
Discharge
Flank pain
MS
Arthralgia
Arthritis
Joint swelling
Myalgias
Back pain
Heme
Bleeding
Bruising
Lymph
Swelling

Endo
Polyuria
Polydypsia
Polyphagia
Derm
Rash
Pruritis
Wound(s)
Neuro
Weakness
Seizures
Parasthesias
Tremors
Syncope
Psych
Anxiety
Depression

+ ROS Findings

PE vitals	HR	BP	RR	T	SPO2	Ht	Wt	BMI%

(check any) **General**	**Neck**	**Pulm**	**Neuro**
( ) No Acute Distress	( ) Midline trachea	( ) No retractions	( ) AAO x 3
( ) Cooperative	( ) nl thyroid w/o	( ) No dullness	( ) CN II-XII intact
( ) nl Hygiene	enlargement	( ) No fremitus	( ) nl sensation
Eyes	( ) No	( ) No wheezing/	( ) Reflexes 2+ &
( ) nl conjunctiva	lymphadenopathy	rales/rhonchi	symmetrical
( ) PERRLA	**CV**	**GI**	( ) nl memory
( ) Size___	( ) PMI	( ) No masses/	( ) nl speech
( ) nl Fundus	nondisplaced	tenderness	**MSK**
( ) nl Discs/vessels	( ) No murmur/	( ) No hep/	( ) nl tone
( ) No scleral icterus	gallop/rub	splenomegaly	( ) nl bulk
ENT	( ) nl intensity w/o	( ) nl bowel sounds	( ) nl gait
( ) No scars/masses	bruit	( ) No dullness	( ) nl ROM UE
( ) nl canals/ TM	( ) No JVD	( ) Heme (-) stool	( ) nl ROM LE
( ) nl hearing bilat	( ) nl femoral/pedal	**GU**	L___/5 UE R___/5
( ) nl teeth/tongue	pulses	( ) nl ext genitalia	L___/5 LE R___/5
	( ) No pedal	( ) No hernia	
	edema		

+ PE Findings

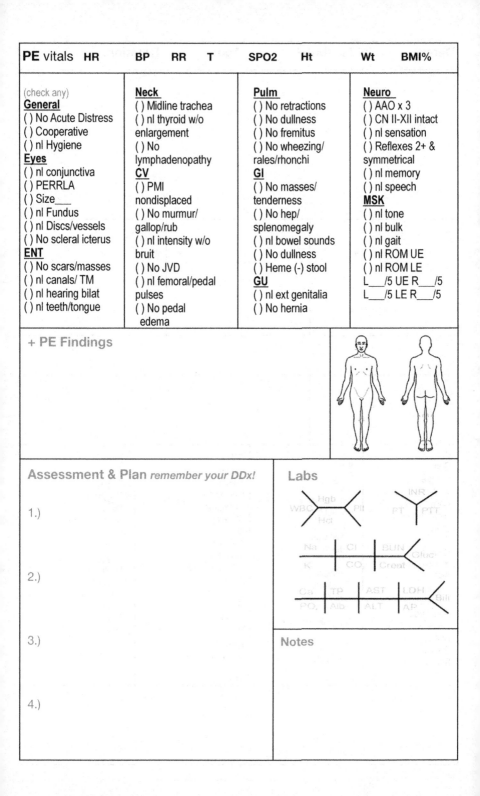

Assessment & Plan *remember your DDx!*

1.)

2.)

3.)

4.)

Labs

Notes

Date:	Initials/MRN:	Age:	Rotation:

CC: _____ y/o M/F
HPI: *symptoms/pertinent +/- ROS/prior episodes/recent travel/sick contacts*

PMHx *child/adult illness /hospitalizations/ immunizations*	**SurgHx** *type/when/ why/complications*	**FamHx** *parents/siblings/ children*

SHx *smoker/ETOH/illicits/exercise/sex/maritalstatus*

Allergies *meds/foods/ environmental/reactions*	**Meds** *reason/dose/time/route/compliance/vitamins/ herbs/otcs*

ROS (circle any)

Gen	**Pulm**	**GU**	**Endo**
Fatigue	Cough	Dysuria	Polyuria
Weight +/-	SOB	Frequency	Polydypsia
Chills	Wheezing	Hematuria	Polyphagia
Night sweats	Hemoptysis	Discharge	**Derm**
Eyes	**CV**	Flank pain	Rash
Pain	Chest pain	**MS**	Pruritis
Redness	Edema	Arthralgia	Wound(s)
Vision changes	PND	Arthritis	**Neuro**
ENT	Orthopnea	Joint swelling	Weakness
Headache	Palpitations	Myalgias	Seizures
Hoarseness	Claudication	Back pain	Parasthesias
Sore throat	**GI**	**Heme**	Tremors
Sinus sx	Abd pain	Bleeding	Syncope
Hearing loss	N/V	Bruising	**Psych**
Tinnitus	Heartburn	**Lymph**	Anxiety
Runny nose	Bloody stools	Swelling	Depression

+ ROS Findings

PE vitals	**HR**	**BP**	**RR**	**T**	**SPO2**	**Ht**	**Wt**	**BMI%**

(check any)

General
( ) No Acute Distress
( ) Cooperative
( ) nl Hygiene

Eyes
( ) nl conjunctiva
( ) PERRLA
( ) Size___
( ) nl Fundus
( ) nl Discs/vessels
( ) No scleral icterus

ENT
( ) No scars/masses
( ) nl canals/ TM
( ) nl hearing bilat
( ) nl teeth/tongue

Neck
( ) Midline trachea
( ) nl thyroid w/o enlargement
( ) No lymphadenopathy

CV
( ) PMI nondisplaced
( ) No murmur/ gallop/rub
( ) nl intensity w/o bruit
( ) No JVD
( ) nl femoral/pedal pulses
( ) No pedal edema

Pulm
( ) No retractions
( ) No dullness
( ) No fremitus
( ) No wheezing/ rales/rhonchi

GI
( ) No masses/ tenderness
( ) No hep/ splenomegaly
( ) nl bowel sounds
( ) No dullness
( ) Heme (-) stool

GU
( ) nl ext genitalia
( ) No hernia

Neuro
( ) AAO x 3
( ) CN II-XII intact
( ) nl sensation
( ) Reflexes 2+ & symmetrical
( ) nl memory
( ) nl speech

MSK
( ) nl tone
( ) nl bulk
( ) nl gait
( ) nl ROM UE
( ) nl ROM LE
L___/5 UE R___/5
L___/5 LE R___/5

+ PE Findings

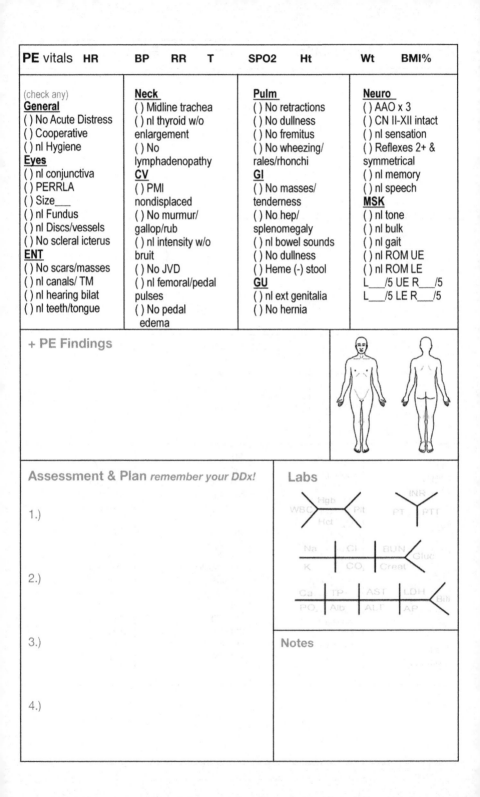

Assessment & Plan *remember your DDx!*

1.)

2.)

3.)

4.)

Labs

Hgb
WBC   Plt
Hct

INR
PT   PTT

Na   Cl   BUN
                              Gluc
K   CO₂   Creat

Ca   TP   AST   LDH
                                    Bili
PO₄   Alb   ALT   AP

Notes

Date:	Initials/MRN:	Age:	Rotation:

CC: _____ y/o M/F
HPI: *symptoms/pertinent +/- ROS/prior episodes/recent travel/sick contacts*

PMHx *child/adult illness /hospitalizations/ immunizations*

SurgHx *type/when/ why/complications*

FamHx *parents/siblings/ children*

SHx *smoker/ETOH/illicits/exercise/sex/maritalstatus*

Allergies *meds/foods/ environmental/reactions*

Meds *reason/dose/time/route/compliance/vitamins/ herbs/otcs*

ROS (circle any)

Gen
Fatigue
Weight +/-
Chills
Night sweats
Eyes
Pain
Redness
Vision changes
ENT
Headache
Hoarseness
Sore throat
Sinus sx
Hearing loss
Tinnitus
Runny nose

Pulm
Cough
SOB
Wheezing
Hemoptysis
CV
Chest pain
Edema
PND
Orthopnea
Palpitations
Claudication
GI
Abd pain
N/V
Heartburn
Bloody stools

GU
Dysuria
Frequency
Hematuria
Discharge
Flank pain
MS
Arthralgia
Arthritis
Joint swelling
Myalgias
Back pain
Heme
Bleeding
Bruising
Lymph
Swelling

Endo
Polyuria
Polydypsia
Polyphagia
Derm
Rash
Pruritis
Wound(s)
Neuro
Weakness
Seizures
Parasthesias
Tremors
Syncope
Psych
Anxiety
Depression

+ ROS Findings

PE vitals   **HR**   **BP**   **RR**   **T**   **SPO2**   **Ht**   **Wt**   **BMI%**

(check any)	**Neck**	**Pulm**	**Neuro**
General	( ) Midline trachea	( ) No retractions	( ) AAO x 3
( ) No Acute Distress	( ) nl thyroid w/o	( ) No dullness	( ) CN II-XII intact
( ) Cooperative	enlargement	( ) No fremitus	( ) nl sensation
( ) nl Hygiene	( ) No	( ) No wheezing/	( ) Reflexes 2+ &
Eyes	lymphadenopathy	rales/rhonchi	symmetrical
( ) nl conjunctiva	**CV**	**GI**	( ) nl memory
( ) PERRLA	( ) PMI	( ) No masses/	( ) nl speech
( ) Size___	nondisplaced	tenderness	**MSK**
( ) nl Fundus	( ) No murmur/	( ) No hep/	( ) nl tone
( ) nl Discs/vessels	gallop/rub	splenomegaly	( ) nl bulk
( ) No scleral icterus	( ) nl intensity w/o	( ) nl bowel sounds	( ) nl gait
ENT	bruit	( ) No dullness	( ) nl ROM UE
( ) No scars/masses	( ) No JVD	( ) Heme (-) stool	( ) nl ROM LE
( ) nl canals/ TM	( ) nl femoral/pedal	**GU**	L___/5 UE R___/5
( ) nl hearing bilat	pulses	( ) nl ext genitalia	L___/5 LE R___/5
( ) nl teeth/tongue	( ) No pedal	( ) No hernia	
	edema		

+ PE Findings

Assessment & Plan *remember your DDx!*

1.)

2.)

3.)

4.)

Labs

Notes

Date: **Initials/MRN:**   **Age:**   **Rotation:**

CC: _____ y/o M/F
HPI: *symptoms/pertinent +/- ROS/prior episodes/recent travel/sick contacts*

PMHx *child/adult illness /hospitalizations/ immunizations*	**SurgHx** *type/when/ why/complications*	**FamHx** *parents/siblings/ children*

SHx *smoker/ETOH/illicits/exercise/sex/maritalstatus*

Allergies *meds/foods/ environmental/reactions*	**Meds** *reason/dose/time/route/compliance/vitamins/ herbs/otcs*

ROS (circle any)

Gen	**Pulm**	**GU**	**Endo**
Fatigue	Cough	Dysuria	Polyuria
Weight +/-	SOB	Frequency	Polydypsia
Chills	Wheezing	Hematuria	Polyphagia
Night sweats	Hemoptysis	Discharge	**Derm**
Eyes	**CV**	Flank pain	Rash
Pain	Chest pain	**MS**	Pruritis
Redness	Edema	Arthralgia	Wound(s)
Vision changes	PND	Arthritis	**Neuro**
ENT	Orthopnea	Joint swelling	Weakness
Headache	Palpitations	Myalgias	Seizures
Hoarseness	Claudication	Back pain	Parasthesias
Sore throat	**GI**	**Heme**	Tremors
Sinus sx	Abd pain	Bleeding	Syncope
Hearing loss	N/V	Bruising	**Psych**
Tinnitus	Heartburn	**Lymph**	Anxiety
Runny nose	Bloody stools	Swelling	Depression

+ ROS Findings

PE vitals HR   BP   RR   T   SPO2   Ht   Wt   BMI%

(check any)	**Neck**	**Pulm**	**Neuro**
General	( ) Midline trachea	( ) No retractions	( ) AAO x 3
( ) No Acute Distress	( ) nl thyroid w/o	( ) No dullness	( ) CN II-XII intact
( ) Cooperative	enlargement	( ) No fremitus	( ) nl sensation
( ) nl Hygiene	( ) No	( ) No wheezing/	( ) Reflexes 2+ &
Eyes	lymphadenopathy	rales/rhonchi	symmetrical
( ) nl conjunctiva	**CV**	**GI**	( ) nl memory
( ) PERRLA	( ) PMI	( ) No masses/	( ) nl speech
( ) Size___	nondisplaced	tenderness	**MSK**
( ) nl Fundus	( ) No murmur/	( ) No hep/	( ) nl tone
( ) nl Discs/vessels	gallop/rub	splenomegaly	( ) nl bulk
( ) No scleral icterus	( ) nl intensity w/o	( ) nl bowel sounds	( ) nl gait
ENT	bruit	( ) No dullness	( ) nl ROM UE
( ) No scars/masses	( ) No JVD	( ) Heme (-) stool	( ) nl ROM LE
( ) nl canals/ TM	( ) nl femoral/pedal	**GU**	L___/5 UE R___/5
( ) nl hearing bilat	pulses	( ) nl ext genitalia	L___/5 LE R___/5
( ) nl teeth/tongue	( ) No pedal	( ) No hernia	
	edema		

+ PE Findings

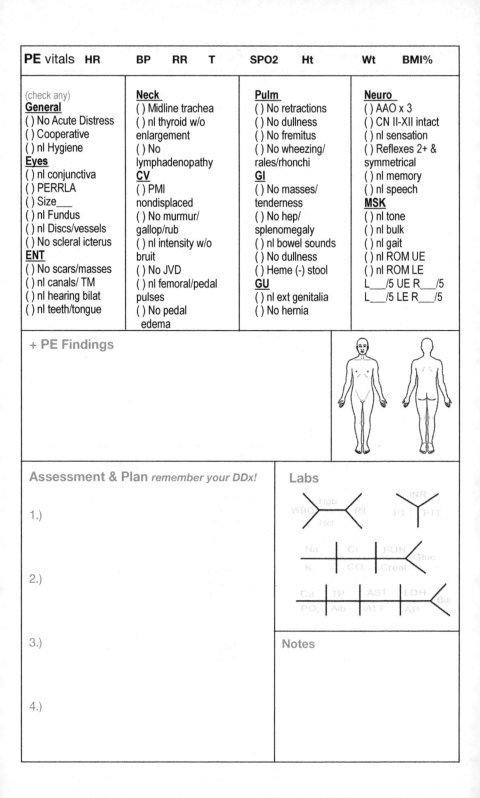

Assessment & Plan *remember your DDx!*

1.)

2.)

3.)

4.)

Labs

WBC Hgb Plt
Hct

Na Cl BUN Gluc
K CO₂ Creat

INR
PT PTT

Ca TP AST LDH Bili
PO₄ Alb ALT AP

Notes

Date:	Initials/MRN:	Age:	Rotation:

CC: _____ y/o M/F
HPI: *symptoms/pertinent +/- ROS/prior episodes/recent travel/sick contacts*

PMHx *child/adult illness /hospitalizations/ immunizations*	**SurgHx** *type/when/ why/complications*	**FamHx** *parents/siblings/ children*

SHx *smoker/ETOH/illicits/exercise/sex/maritalstatus*

Allergies *meds/foods/ environmental/reactions*	**Meds** *reason/dose/time/route/compliance/vitamins/ herbs/otcs*

ROS (circle any)

Gen	**Pulm**	**GU**	**Endo**
Fatigue	Cough	Dysuria	Polyuria
Weight +/-	SOB	Frequency	Polydypsia
Chills	Wheezing	Hematuria	Polyphagia
Night sweats	Hemoptysis	Discharge	**Derm**
Eyes	**CV**	Flank pain	Rash
Pain	Chest pain	**MS**	Pruritis
Redness	Edema	Arthralgia	Wound(s)
Vision changes	PND	Arthritis	**Neuro**
ENT	Orthopnea	Joint swelling	Weakness
Headache	Palpitations	Myalgias	Seizures
Hoarseness	Claudication	Back pain	Parasthesias
Sore throat	**GI**	**Heme**	Tremors
Sinus sx	Abd pain	Bleeding	Syncope
Hearing loss	N/V	Bruising	**Psych**
Tinnitus	Heartburn	**Lymph**	Anxiety
Runny nose	Bloody stools	Swelling	Depression

+ ROS Findings

PE vitals   **HR**   **BP**   **RR**   **T**   **SPO2**   **Ht**   **Wt**   **BMI%**

(check any)	**Neck**	**Pulm**	**Neuro**
General	( ) Midline trachea	( ) No retractions	( ) AAO x 3
( ) No Acute Distress	( ) nl thyroid w/o	( ) No dullness	( ) CN II-XII intact
( ) Cooperative	enlargement	( ) No fremitus	( ) nl sensation
( ) nl Hygiene	( ) No	( ) No wheezing/	( ) Reflexes 2+ &
Eyes	lymphadenopathy	rales/rhonchi	symmetrical
( ) nl conjunctiva	**CV**	**GI**	( ) nl memory
( ) PERRLA	( ) PMI	( ) No masses/	( ) nl speech
( ) Size___	nondisplaced	tenderness	**MSK**
( ) nl Fundus	( ) No murmur/	( ) No hep/	( ) nl tone
( ) nl Discs/vessels	gallop/rub	splenomegaly	( ) nl bulk
( ) No scleral icterus	( ) nl intensity w/o	( ) nl bowel sounds	( ) nl gait
ENT	bruit	( ) No dullness	( ) nl ROM UE
( ) No scars/masses	( ) No JVD	( ) Heme (-) stool	( ) nl ROM LE
( ) nl canals/ TM	( ) nl femoral/pedal	**GU**	L___/5 UE R___/5
( ) nl hearing bilat	pulses	( ) nl ext genitalia	L___/5 LE R___/5
( ) nl teeth/tongue	( ) No pedal	( ) No hernia	
	edema		

+ PE Findings

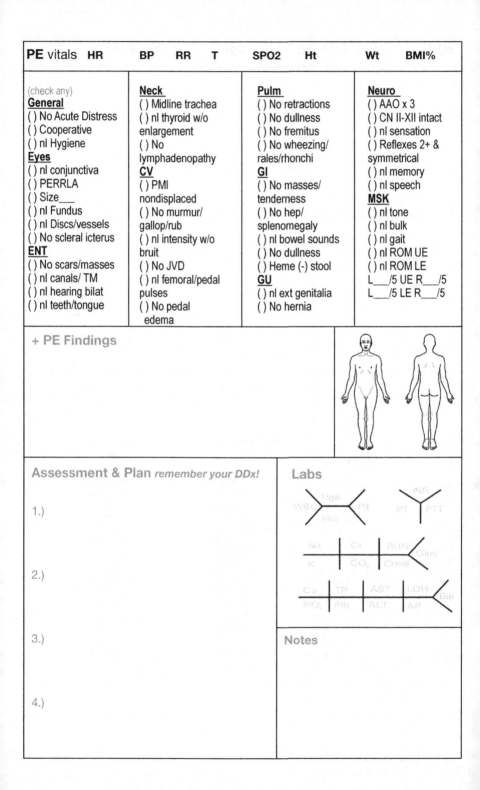

Assessment & Plan *remember your DDx!*

1.)

2.)

3.)

4.)

Labs

Notes

Date:	Initials/MRN:	Age:	Rotation:

CC: _____ y/o M/F
HPI: *symptoms/pertinent +/- ROS/prior episodes/recent travel/sick contacts*

PMHx *child/adult illness /hospitalizations/ immunizations*

SurgHx *type/when/ why/complications*

FamHx *parents/siblings/ children*

SHx *smoker/ETOH/illicits/exercise/sex/maritalstatus*

Allergies *meds/foods/ environmental/reactions*

Meds *reason/dose/time/route/compliance/vitamins/ herbs/otcs*

ROS (circle any)

Gen
Fatigue
Weight +/-
Chills
Night sweats
Eyes
Pain
Redness
Vision changes
ENT
Headache
Hoarseness
Sore throat
Sinus sx
Hearing loss
Tinnitus
Runny nose

Pulm
Cough
SOB
Wheezing
Hemoptysis
CV
Chest pain
Edema
PND
Orthopnea
Palpitations
Claudication
GI
Abd pain
N/V
Heartburn
Bloody stools

GU
Dysuria
Frequency
Hematuria
Discharge
Flank pain
MS
Arthralgia
Arthritis
Joint swelling
Myalgias
Back pain
Heme
Bleeding
Bruising
Lymph
Swelling

Endo
Polyuria
Polydypsia
Polyphagia
Derm
Rash
Pruritis
Wound(s)
Neuro
Weakness
Seizures
Parasthesias
Tremors
Syncope
Psych
Anxiety
Depression

+ ROS Findings

PE vitals   **HR**   **BP**   **RR**   **T**   **SPO2**   **Ht**   **Wt**   **BMI%**

(check any)	**Neck**	**Pulm**	**Neuro**
General	( ) Midline trachea	( ) No retractions	( ) AAO x 3
( ) No Acute Distress	( ) nl thyroid w/o	( ) No dullness	( ) CN II-XII intact
( ) Cooperative	enlargement	( ) No fremitus	( ) nl sensation
( ) nl Hygiene	( ) No	( ) No wheezing/	( ) Reflexes 2+ &
Eyes	lymphadenopathy	rales/rhonchi	symmetrical
( ) nl conjunctiva	**CV**	**GI**	( ) nl memory
( ) PERRLA	( ) PMI	( ) No masses/	( ) nl speech
( ) Size___	nondisplaced	tenderness	**MSK**
( ) nl Fundus	( ) No murmur/	( ) No hep/	( ) nl tone
( ) nl Discs/vessels	gallop/rub	splenomegaly	( ) nl bulk
( ) No scleral icterus	( ) nl intensity w/o	( ) nl bowel sounds	( ) nl gait
ENT	bruit	( ) No dullness	( ) nl ROM UE
( ) No scars/masses	( ) No JVD	( ) Heme (-) stool	( ) nl ROM LE
( ) nl canals/ TM	( ) nl femoral/pedal	**GU**	L___/5 UE R___/5
( ) nl hearing bilat	pulses	( ) nl ext genitalia	L___/5 LE R___/5
( ) nl teeth/tongue	( ) No pedal	( ) No hernia	
	edema		

+ PE Findings

Assessment & Plan *remember your DDx!*

1.)

2.)

3.)

4.)

Labs

Notes

Date:	Initials/MRN:	Age:	Rotation:

CC: _____ y/o M/F
HPI: *symptoms/pertinent +/- ROS/prior episodes/recent travel/sick contacts*

PMHx *child/adult illness /hospitalizations/ immunizations*

SurgHx *type/when/ why/complications*

FamHx *parents/siblings/ children*

SHx *smoker/ETOH/illicits/exercise/sex/maritalstatus*

Allergies *meds/foods/ environmental/reactions*

Meds *reason/dose/time/route/compliance/vitamins/ herbs/otcs*

ROS (circle any)

Gen
Fatigue
Weight +/-
Chills
Night sweats
Eyes
Pain
Redness
Vision changes
ENT
Headache
Hoarseness
Sore throat
Sinus sx
Hearing loss
Tinnitus
Runny nose

Pulm
Cough
SOB
Wheezing
Hemoptysis
CV
Chest pain
Edema
PND
Orthopnea
Palpitations
Claudication
GI
Abd pain
N/V
Heartburn
Bloody stools

GU
Dysuria
Frequency
Hematuria
Discharge
Flank pain
MS
Arthralgia
Arthritis
Joint swelling
Myalgias
Back pain
Heme
Bleeding
Bruising
Lymph
Swelling

Endo
Polyuria
Polydypsia
Polyphagia
Derm
Rash
Pruritis
Wound(s)
Neuro
Weakness
Seizures
Parasthesias
Tremors
Syncope
Psych
Anxiety
Depression

+ ROS Findings

PE vitals	HR	BP	RR	T	SPO2	Ht	Wt	BMI%

(check any)	**Neck**	**Pulm**	**Neuro**
General	( ) Midline trachea	( ) No retractions	( ) AAO x 3
( ) No Acute Distress	( ) nl thyroid w/o	( ) No dullness	( ) CN II-XII intact
( ) Cooperative	enlargement	( ) No fremitus	( ) nl sensation
( ) nl Hygiene	( ) No	( ) No wheezing/	( ) Reflexes 2+ &
Eyes	lymphadenopathy	rales/rhonchi	symmetrical
( ) nl conjunctiva	**CV**	**GI**	( ) nl memory
( ) PERRLA	( ) PMI	( ) No masses/	( ) nl speech
( ) Size___	nondisplaced	tenderness	**MSK**
( ) nl Fundus	( ) No murmur/	( ) No hep/	( ) nl tone
( ) nl Discs/vessels	gallop/rub	splenomegaly	( ) nl bulk
( ) No scleral icterus	( ) nl intensity w/o	( ) nl bowel sounds	( ) nl gait
ENT	bruit	( ) No dullness	( ) nl ROM UE
( ) No scars/masses	( ) No JVD	( ) Heme (-) stool	( ) nl ROM LE
( ) nl canals/ TM	( ) nl femoral/pedal	**GU**	L___/5 UE R___/5
( ) nl hearing bilat	pulses	( ) nl ext genitalia	L___/5 LE R___/5
( ) nl teeth/tongue	( ) No pedal	( ) No hernia	
	edema		

+ PE Findings

Assessment & Plan *remember your DDx!*

1.)

2.)

3.)

4.)

Labs

Hgb
WBC — Plt
Hct

INR
PT — PTT

Na | Cl | BUN
K | CO₂ | Creat — Gluc

Ca | TP | AST | LDH
PO₄ | Alb | ALT | AP — Bili

Notes

Date:　　　　**Initials/MRN:**　　　　**Age:**　　　　**Rotation:**

CC: _____ y/o M/F
HPI: *symptoms/pertinent +/- ROS/prior episodes/recent travel/sick contacts*

PMHx *child/adult illness /hospitalizations/ immunizations*

SurgHx *type/when/ why/complications*

FamHx *parents/siblings/ children*

SHx *smoker/ETOH/illicits/exercise/sex/maritalstatus*

Allergies *meds/foods/ environmental/reactions*

Meds *reason/dose/time/route/compliance/vitamins/ herbs/otcs*

ROS (circle any)

Gen
Fatigue
Weight +/-
Chills
Night sweats
Eyes
Pain
Redness
Vision changes
ENT
Headache
Hoarseness
Sore throat
Sinus sx
Hearing loss
Tinnitus
Runny nose

Pulm
Cough
SOB
Wheezing
Hemoptysis
CV
Chest pain
Edema
PND
Orthopnea
Palpitations
Claudication
GI
Abd pain
N/V
Heartburn
Bloody stools

GU
Dysuria
Frequency
Hematuria
Discharge
Flank pain
MS
Arthralgia
Arthritis
Joint swelling
Myalgias
Back pain
Heme
Bleeding
Bruising
Lymph
Swelling

Endo
Polyuria
Polydypsia
Polyphagia
Derm
Rash
Pruritis
Wound(s)
Neuro
Weakness
Seizures
Parasthesias
Tremors
Syncope
Psych
Anxiety
Depression

+ ROS Findings

PE vitals   **HR**   **BP**   **RR**   **T**   **SPO2**   **Ht**   **Wt**   **BMI%**

(check any)	**Neck**	**Pulm**	**Neuro**
General	( ) Midline trachea	( ) No retractions	( ) AAO x 3
( ) No Acute Distress	( ) nl thyroid w/o	( ) No dullness	( ) CN II-XII intact
( ) Cooperative	enlargement	( ) No fremitus	( ) nl sensation
( ) nl Hygiene	( ) No	( ) No wheezing/	( ) Reflexes 2+ &
Eyes	lymphadenopathy	rales/rhonchi	symmetrical
( ) nl conjunctiva	**CV**	**GI**	( ) nl memory
( ) PERRLA	( ) PMI	( ) No masses/	( ) nl speech
( ) Size___	nondisplaced	tenderness	**MSK**
( ) nl Fundus	( ) No murmur/	( ) No hep/	( ) nl tone
( ) nl Discs/vessels	gallop/rub	splenomegaly	( ) nl bulk
( ) No scleral icterus	( ) nl intensity w/o	( ) nl bowel sounds	( ) nl gait
ENT	bruit	( ) No dullness	( ) nl ROM UE
( ) No scars/masses	( ) No JVD	( ) Heme (-) stool	( ) nl ROM LE
( ) nl canals/ TM	( ) nl femoral/pedal	**GU**	L___/5 UE R___/5
( ) nl hearing bilat	pulses	( ) nl ext genitalia	L___/5 LE R___/5
( ) nl teeth/tongue	( ) No pedal	( ) No hernia	
	edema		

+ PE Findings

Assessment & Plan *remember your DDx!*

1.)

2.)

3.)

4.)

Labs

Notes

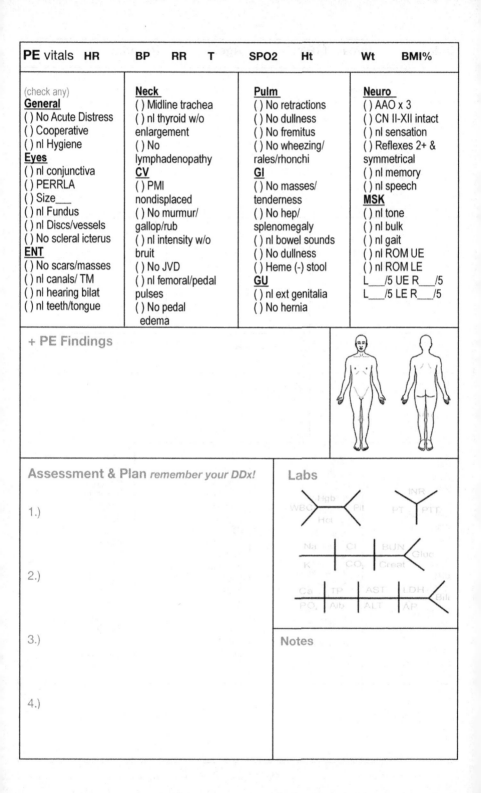

Date:	Initials/MRN:	Age:	Rotation:

CC: _____ y/o M/F
HPI: *symptoms/pertinent +/- ROS/prior episodes/recent travel/sick contacts*

PMHx *child/adult illness /hospitalizations/ immunizations*	**SurgHx** *type/when/ why/complications*	**FamHx** *parents/siblings/ children*

SHx *smoker/ETOH/illicits/exercise/sex/maritalstatus*

Allergies *meds/foods/ environmental/reactions*	**Meds** *reason/dose/time/route/compliance/vitamins/ herbs/otcs*

ROS (circle any)

Gen	**Pulm**	**GU**	**Endo**
Fatigue	Cough	Dysuria	Polyuria
Weight +/-	SOB	Frequency	Polydypsia
Chills	Wheezing	Hematuria	Polyphagia
Night sweats	Hemoptysis	Discharge	**Derm**
Eyes	**CV**	Flank pain	Rash
Pain	Chest pain	**MS**	Pruritis
Redness	Edema	Arthralgia	Wound(s)
Vision changes	PND	Arthritis	**Neuro**
ENT	Orthopnea	Joint swelling	Weakness
Headache	Palpitations	Myalgias	Seizures
Hoarseness	Claudication	Back pain	Parasthesias
Sore throat	**GI**	**Heme**	Tremors
Sinus sx	Abd pain	Bleeding	Syncope
Hearing loss	N/V	Bruising	**Psych**
Tinnitus	Heartburn	**Lymph**	Anxiety
Runny nose	Bloody stools	Swelling	Depression

+ ROS Findings

PE vitals HR	BP	RR	T	SPO2	Ht	Wt	BMI%

(check any)	**Neck**	**Pulm**	**Neuro**
General	( ) Midline trachea	( ) No retractions	( ) AAO x 3
( ) No Acute Distress	( ) nl thyroid w/o	( ) No dullness	( ) CN II-XII intact
( ) Cooperative	enlargement	( ) No fremitus	( ) nl sensation
( ) nl Hygiene	( ) No	( ) No wheezing/	( ) Reflexes 2+ &
Eyes	lymphadenopathy	rales/rhonchi	symmetrical
( ) nl conjunctiva	**CV**	**GI**	( ) nl memory
( ) PERRLA	( ) PMI	( ) No masses/	( ) nl speech
( ) Size___	nondisplaced	tenderness	**MSK**
( ) nl Fundus	( ) No murmur/	( ) No hep/	( ) nl tone
( ) nl Discs/vessels	gallop/rub	splenomegaly	( ) nl bulk
( ) No scleral icterus	( ) nl intensity w/o	( ) nl bowel sounds	( ) nl gait
ENT	bruit	( ) No dullness	( ) nl ROM UE
( ) No scars/masses	( ) No JVD	( ) Heme (-) stool	( ) nl ROM LE
( ) nl canals/ TM	( ) nl femoral/pedal	**GU**	L___/5 UE R___/5
( ) nl hearing bilat	pulses	( ) nl ext genitalia	L___/5 LE R___/5
( ) nl teeth/tongue	( ) No pedal	( ) No hernia	
	edema		

+ PE Findings

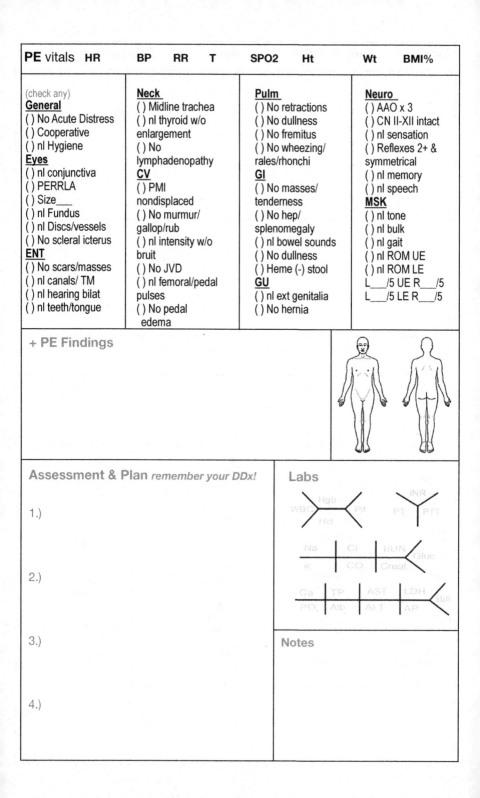

Assessment & Plan *remember your DDx!*

1.)

2.)

3.)

4.)

Labs

Hgb
WBC   Plt
Hct

INR
PT   PTT

Na   Cl   BUN
K   CO₂   Creat   Gluc

Ca   TP   AST   LDH
PO₄   Alb   ALT   AP   Bili

Notes

Date:	Initials/MRN:	Age:	Rotation:

CC: _____ y/o M/F
HPI: *symptoms/pertinent +/- ROS/prior episodes/recent travel/sick contacts*

PMHx *child/adult illness /hospitalizations/ immunizations*	**SurgHx** *type/when/ why/complications*	**FamHx** *parents/siblings/ children*

SHx *smoker/ETOH/illicits/exercise/sex/maritalstatus*

Allergies *meds/foods/ environmental/reactions*	**Meds** *reason/dose/time/route/compliance/vitamins/ herbs/otcs*

ROS (circle any)

Gen	**Pulm**	**GU**	**Endo**
Fatigue	Cough	Dysuria	Polyuria
Weight +/-	SOB	Frequency	Polydypsia
Chills	Wheezing	Hematuria	Polyphagia
Night sweats	Hemoptysis	Discharge	**Derm**
Eyes	**CV**	Flank pain	Rash
Pain	Chest pain	**MS**	Pruritis
Redness	Edema	Arthralgia	Wound(s)
Vision changes	PND	Arthritis	**Neuro**
ENT	Orthopnea	Joint swelling	Weakness
Headache	Palpitations	Myalgias	Seizures
Hoarseness	Claudication	Back pain	Parasthesias
Sore throat	**GI**	**Heme**	Tremors
Sinus sx	Abd pain	Bleeding	Syncope
Hearing loss	N/V	Bruising	**Psych**
Tinnitus	Heartburn	**Lymph**	Anxiety
Runny nose	Bloody stools	Swelling	Depression

+ ROS Findings

PE vitals **HR**	**BP**	**RR**	**T**	**SPO2**	**Ht**	**Wt**	**BMI%**

(check any)

General
( ) No Acute Distress
( ) Cooperative
( ) nl Hygiene
Eyes
( ) nl conjunctiva
( ) PERRLA
( ) Size___
( ) nl Fundus
( ) nl Discs/vessels
( ) No scleral icterus
ENT
( ) No scars/masses
( ) nl canals/ TM
( ) nl hearing bilat
( ) nl teeth/tongue

Neck
( ) Midline trachea
( ) nl thyroid w/o
enlargement
( ) No
lymphadenopathy
CV
( ) PMI
nondisplaced
( ) No murmur/
gallop/rub
( ) nl intensity w/o
bruit
( ) No JVD
( ) nl femoral/pedal
pulses
( ) No pedal
edema

Pulm
( ) No retractions
( ) No dullness
( ) No fremitus
( ) No wheezing/
rales/rhonchi
GI
( ) No masses/
tenderness
( ) No hep/
splenomegaly
( ) nl bowel sounds
( ) No dullness
( ) Heme (-) stool
GU
( ) nl ext genitalia
( ) No hernia

Neuro
( ) AAO x 3
( ) CN II-XII intact
( ) nl sensation
( ) Reflexes 2+ &
symmetrical
( ) nl memory
( ) nl speech
MSK
( ) nl tone
( ) nl bulk
( ) nl gait
( ) nl ROM UE
( ) nl ROM LE
L___/5 UE R___/5
L___/5 LE R___/5

+ PE Findings

Assessment & Plan *remember your DDx!*

1.)

2.)

3.)

4.)

Labs

Hgb
WBC   Plt
Hct

INR
PT   PTT

Na   Cl   BUN
                     Gluc
K   CO₂   Creat

Ca   TP   AST   LDH
                            Bili
PO₄ Alb   ALT   AP

Notes

Date:	Initials/MRN:	Age:	Rotation:

CC: _____ y/o M/F
HPI: *symptoms/pertinent +/- ROS/prior episodes/recent travel/sick contacts*

PMHx *child/adult illness /hospitalizations/ immunizations*	**SurgHx** *type/when/ why/complications*	**FamHx** *parents/siblings/ children*

SHx *smoker/ETOH/illicits/exercise/sex/maritalstatus*

Allergies *meds/foods/ environmental/reactions*	**Meds** *reason/dose/time/route/compliance/vitamins/ herbs/otcs*

ROS (circle any)

Gen	**Pulm**	**GU**	**Endo**
Fatigue	Cough	Dysuria	Polyuria
Weight +/-	SOB	Frequency	Polydypsia
Chills	Wheezing	Hematuria	Polyphagia
Night sweats	Hemoptysis	Discharge	**Derm**
Eyes	**CV**	Flank pain	Rash
Pain	Chest pain	**MS**	Pruritis
Redness	Edema	Arthralgia	Wound(s)
Vision changes	PND	Arthritis	**Neuro**
ENT	Orthopnea	Joint swelling	Weakness
Headache	Palpitations	Myalgias	Seizures
Hoarseness	Claudication	Back pain	Parasthesias
Sore throat	**GI**	**Heme**	Tremors
Sinus sx	Abd pain	Bleeding	Syncope
Hearing loss	N/V	Bruising	**Psych**
Tinnitus	Heartburn	**Lymph**	Anxiety
Runny nose	Bloody stools	Swelling	Depression

+ ROS Findings

PE vitals	**HR**	**BP**	**RR**	**T**	**SPO2**	**Ht**	**Wt**	**BMI%**

(check any)

General
( ) No Acute Distress
( ) Cooperative
( ) nl Hygiene
Eyes
( ) nl conjunctiva
( ) PERRLA
( ) Size___
( ) nl Fundus
( ) nl Discs/vessels
( ) No scleral icterus
ENT
( ) No scars/masses
( ) nl canals/ TM
( ) nl hearing bilat
( ) nl teeth/tongue

Neck
( ) Midline trachea
( ) nl thyroid w/o
enlargement
( ) No
lymphadenopathy
CV
( ) PMI
nondisplaced
( ) No murmur/
gallop/rub
( ) nl intensity w/o
bruit
( ) No JVD
( ) nl femoral/pedal
pulses
( ) No pedal
edema

Pulm
( ) No retractions
( ) No dullness
( ) No fremitus
( ) No wheezing/
rales/rhonchi
GI
( ) No masses/
tenderness
( ) No hep/
splenomegaly
( ) nl bowel sounds
( ) No dullness
( ) Heme (-) stool
GU
( ) nl ext genitalia
( ) No hernia

Neuro
( ) AAO x 3
( ) CN II-XII intact
( ) nl sensation
( ) Reflexes 2+ &
symmetrical
( ) nl memory
( ) nl speech
MSK
( ) nl tone
( ) nl bulk
( ) nl gait
( ) nl ROM UE
( ) nl ROM LE
L___/5 UE R___/5
L___/5 LE R___/5

+ PE Findings

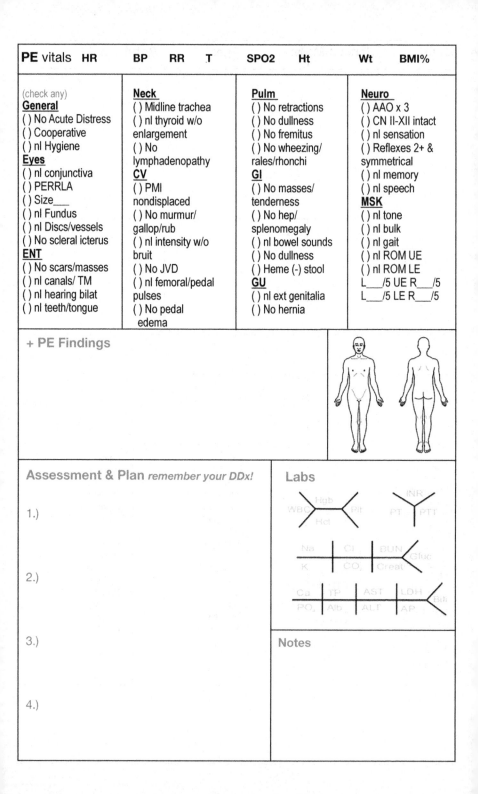

Assessment & Plan *remember your DDx!*

1.)

2.)

3.)

4.)

Labs

WBC / Hgb \ Plt
Hct

INR
PT / \ PTT

Na | Cl | BUN \ Gluc
K | CO₂ | Creat

Ca | TP | AST | LDH \ Bili
PO₄ | Alb | ALT | AP

Notes

Date:	Initials/MRN:	Age:	Rotation:

CC: _____ y/o M/F
HPI: *symptoms/pertinent +/- ROS/prior episodes/recent travel/sick contacts*

PMHx *child/adult illness /hospitalizations/ immunizations*	**SurgHx** *type/when/ why/complications*	**FamHx** *parents/siblings/ children*

SHx *smoker/ETOH/illicits/exercise/sex/maritalstatus*

Allergies *meds/foods/ environmental/reactions*	**Meds** *reason/dose/time/route/compliance/vitamins/ herbs/otcs*

ROS (circle any)

Gen	**Pulm**	**GU**	**Endo**
Fatigue	Cough	Dysuria	Polyuria
Weight +/-	SOB	Frequency	Polydypsia
Chills	Wheezing	Hematuria	Polyphagia
Night sweats	Hemoptysis	Discharge	**Derm**
Eyes	**CV**	Flank pain	Rash
Pain	Chest pain	**MS**	Pruritis
Redness	Edema	Arthralgia	Wound(s)
Vision changes	PND	Arthritis	**Neuro**
ENT	Orthopnea	Joint swelling	Weakness
Headache	Palpitations	Myalgias	Seizures
Hoarseness	Claudication	Back pain	Parasthesias
Sore throat	**GI**	**Heme**	Tremors
Sinus sx	Abd pain	Bleeding	Syncope
Hearing loss	N/V	Bruising	**Psych**
Tinnitus	Heartburn	**Lymph**	Anxiety
Runny nose	Bloody stools	Swelling	Depression

+ ROS Findings

PE vitals	**HR**	**BP**	**RR**	**T**	**SPO2**	**Ht**	**Wt**	**BMI%**

(check any)

General
( ) No Acute Distress
( ) Cooperative
( ) nl Hygiene

Eyes
( ) nl conjunctiva
( ) PERRLA
( ) Size___
( ) nl Fundus
( ) nl Discs/vessels
( ) No scleral icterus

ENT
( ) No scars/masses
( ) nl canals/ TM
( ) nl hearing bilat
( ) nl teeth/tongue

Neck
( ) Midline trachea
( ) nl thyroid w/o
enlargement
( ) No
lymphadenopathy

CV
( ) PMI
nondisplaced
( ) No murmur/
gallop/rub
( ) nl intensity w/o
bruit
( ) No JVD
( ) nl femoral/pedal
pulses
( ) No pedal
edema

Pulm
( ) No retractions
( ) No dullness
( ) No fremitus
( ) No wheezing/
rales/rhonchi

GI
( ) No masses/
tenderness
( ) No hep/
splenomegaly
( ) nl bowel sounds
( ) No dullness
( ) Heme (-) stool

GU
( ) nl ext genitalia
( ) No hernia

Neuro
( ) AAO x 3
( ) CN II-XII intact
( ) nl sensation
( ) Reflexes 2+ &
symmetrical
( ) nl memory
( ) nl speech

MSK
( ) nl tone
( ) nl bulk
( ) nl gait
( ) nl ROM UE
( ) nl ROM LE
L___/5 UE R___/5
L___/5 LE R___/5

+ PE Findings

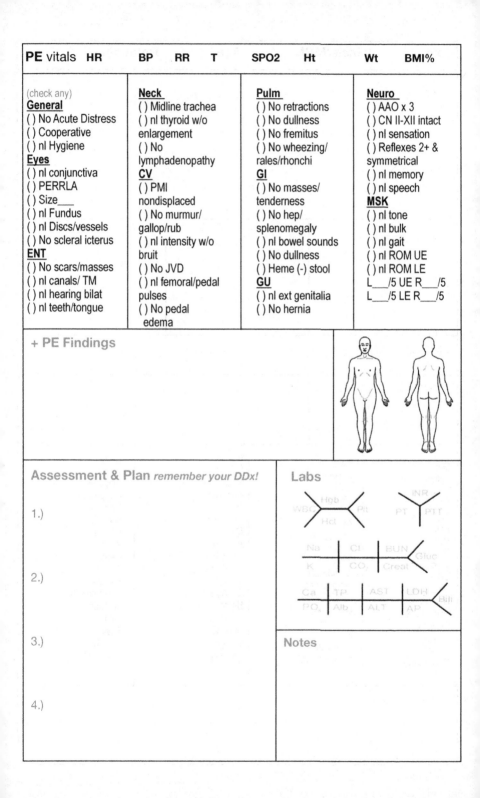

Assessment & Plan *remember your DDx!*

1.)

2.)

3.)

4.)

Labs

Hgb
WBC   Plt
Hct

INR
PT   PTT

Na   Cl   BUN
Gluc
K   CO₂   Creat

Ca   TP   AST   LDH
Bili
PO₄   Alb   ALT   AP

Notes

Date:	Initials/MRN:	Age:	Rotation:

CC: _____ y/o M/F
HPI: *symptoms/pertinent +/- ROS/prior episodes/recent travel/sick contacts*

PMHx *child/adult illness /hospitalizations/ immunizations*	**SurgHx** *type/when/ why/complications*	**FamHx** *parents/siblings/ children*

SHx *smoker/ETOH/illicits/exercise/sex/maritalstatus*

Allergies *meds/foods/ environmental/reactions*	**Meds** *reason/dose/time/route/compliance/vitamins/ herbs/otcs*

ROS (circle any)

Gen	**Pulm**	**GU**	**Endo**
Fatigue	Cough	Dysuria	Polyuria
Weight +/-	SOB	Frequency	Polydypsia
Chills	Wheezing	Hematuria	Polyphagia
Night sweats	Hemoptysis	Discharge	**Derm**
Eyes	**CV**	Flank pain	Rash
Pain	Chest pain	**MS**	Pruritis
Redness	Edema	Arthralgia	Wound(s)
Vision changes	PND	Arthritis	**Neuro**
ENT	Orthopnea	Joint swelling	Weakness
Headache	Palpitations	Myalgias	Seizures
Hoarseness	Claudication	Back pain	Parasthesias
Sore throat	**GI**	**Heme**	Tremors
Sinus sx	Abd pain	Bleeding	Syncope
Hearing loss	N/V	Bruising	**Psych**
Tinnitus	Heartburn	**Lymph**	Anxiety
Runny nose	Bloody stools	Swelling	Depression

+ ROS Findings

PE vitals HR	BP	RR	T	SPO2	Ht	Wt	BMI%

(check any)	**Neck**	**Pulm**	**Neuro**
General	( ) Midline trachea	( ) No retractions	( ) AAO x 3
( ) No Acute Distress	( ) nl thyroid w/o	( ) No dullness	( ) CN II-XII intact
( ) Cooperative	enlargement	( ) No fremitus	( ) nl sensation
( ) nl Hygiene	( ) No	( ) No wheezing/	( ) Reflexes 2+ &
Eyes	lymphadenopathy	rales/rhonchi	symmetrical
( ) nl conjunctiva	**CV**	**GI**	( ) nl memory
( ) PERRLA	( ) PMI	( ) No masses/	( ) nl speech
( ) Size___	nondisplaced	tenderness	**MSK**
( ) nl Fundus	( ) No murmur/	( ) No hep/	( ) nl tone
( ) nl Discs/vessels	gallop/rub	splenomegaly	( ) nl bulk
( ) No scleral icterus	( ) nl intensity w/o	( ) nl bowel sounds	( ) nl gait
ENT	bruit	( ) No dullness	( ) nl ROM UE
( ) No scars/masses	( ) No JVD	( ) Heme (-) stool	( ) nl ROM LE
( ) nl canals/ TM	( ) nl femoral/pedal	**GU**	L___/5 UE R___/5
( ) nl hearing bilat	pulses	( ) nl ext genitalia	L___/5 LE R___/5
( ) nl teeth/tongue	( ) No pedal	( ) No hernia	
	edema		

+ PE Findings

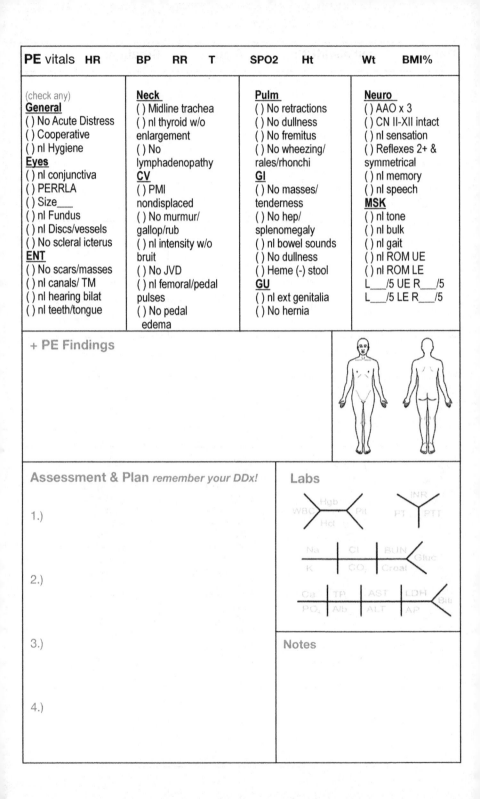

Assessment & Plan *remember your DDx!*

1.)

2.)

3.)

4.)

Labs

Notes

Date:	Initials/MRN:	Age:	Rotation:

CC: _____ y/o M/F
HPI: *symptoms/pertinent +/- ROS/prior episodes/recent travel/sick contacts*

PMHx *child/adult illness /hospitalizations/ immunizations*

SurgHx *type/when/ why/complications*

FamHx *parents/siblings/ children*

SHx *smoker/ETOH/illicits/exercise/sex/maritalstatus*

Allergies *meds/foods/ environmental/reactions*

Meds *reason/dose/time/route/compliance/vitamins/ herbs/otcs*

ROS (circle any)

Gen
Fatigue
Weight +/-
Chills
Night sweats
Eyes
Pain
Redness
Vision changes
ENT
Headache
Hoarseness
Sore throat
Sinus sx
Hearing loss
Tinnitus
Runny nose

Pulm
Cough
SOB
Wheezing
Hemoptysis
CV
Chest pain
Edema
PND
Orthopnea
Palpitations
Claudication
GI
Abd pain
N/V
Heartburn
Bloody stools

GU
Dysuria
Frequency
Hematuria
Discharge
Flank pain
MS
Arthralgia
Arthritis
Joint swelling
Myalgias
Back pain
Heme
Bleeding
Bruising
Lymph
Swelling

Endo
Polyuria
Polydypsia
Polyphagia
Derm
Rash
Pruritis
Wound(s)
Neuro
Weakness
Seizures
Parasthesias
Tremors
Syncope
Psych
Anxiety
Depression

+ **ROS Findings**

PE vitals   **HR**   **BP**   **RR**   **T**   **SPO2**   **Ht**   **Wt**   **BMI%**

(check any)	**Neck**	**Pulm**	**Neuro**
General	( ) Midline trachea	( ) No retractions	( ) AAO x 3
( ) No Acute Distress	( ) nl thyroid w/o	( ) No dullness	( ) CN II-XII intact
( ) Cooperative	enlargement	( ) No fremitus	( ) nl sensation
( ) nl Hygiene	( ) No	( ) No wheezing/	( ) Reflexes 2+ &
Eyes	lymphadenopathy	rales/rhonchi	symmetrical
( ) nl conjunctiva	**CV**	**GI**	( ) nl memory
( ) PERRLA	( ) PMI	( ) No masses/	( ) nl speech
( ) Size___	nondisplaced	tenderness	**MSK**
( ) nl Fundus	( ) No murmur/	( ) No hep/	( ) nl tone
( ) nl Discs/vessels	gallop/rub	splenomegaly	( ) nl bulk
( ) No scleral icterus	( ) nl intensity w/o	( ) nl bowel sounds	( ) nl gait
ENT	bruit	( ) No dullness	( ) nl ROM UE
( ) No scars/masses	( ) No JVD	( ) Heme (-) stool	( ) nl ROM LE
( ) nl canals/ TM	( ) nl femoral/pedal	**GU**	L___/5 UE R___/5
( ) nl hearing bilat	pulses	( ) nl ext genitalia	L___/5 LE R___/5
( ) nl teeth/tongue	( ) No pedal	( ) No hernia	
	edema		

+ PE Findings

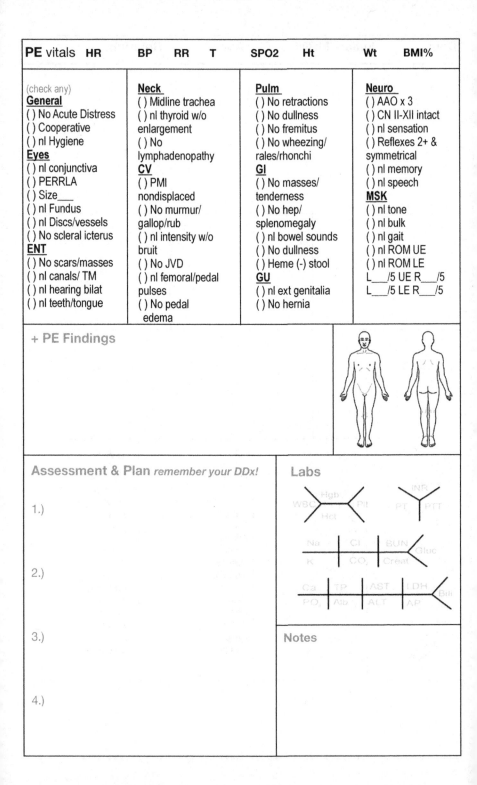

Assessment & Plan *remember your DDx!*

1.)

2.)

3.)

4.)

Labs

Notes

Date:	Initials/MRN:	Age:	Rotation:

CC: _____ y/o M/F
HPI: *symptoms/pertinent +/- ROS/prior episodes/recent travel/sick contacts*

PMHx *child/adult illness /hospitalizations/ immunizations*

SurgHx *type/when/ why/complications*

FamHx *parents/siblings/ children*

SHx *smoker/ETOH/illicits/exercise/sex/maritalstatus*

Allergies *meds/foods/ environmental/reactions*

Meds *reason/dose/time/route/compliance/vitamins/ herbs/otcs*

ROS (circle any)

Gen
Fatigue
Weight +/-
Chills
Night sweats
Eyes
Pain
Redness
Vision changes
ENT
Headache
Hoarseness
Sore throat
Sinus sx
Hearing loss
Tinnitus
Runny nose

Pulm
Cough
SOB
Wheezing
Hemoptysis
CV
Chest pain
Edema
PND
Orthopnea
Palpitations
Claudication
GI
Abd pain
N/V
Heartburn
Bloody stools

GU
Dysuria
Frequency
Hematuria
Discharge
Flank pain
MS
Arthralgia
Arthritis
Joint swelling
Myalgias
Back pain
Heme
Bleeding
Bruising
Lymph
Swelling

Endo
Polyuria
Polydypsia
Polyphagia
Derm
Rash
Pruritis
Wound(s)
Neuro
Weakness
Seizures
Parasthesias
Tremors
Syncope
Psych
Anxiety
Depression

+ ROS Findings

PE vitals   HR   BP   RR   T   SPO2   Ht   Wt   BMI%

(check any)	**Neck**	**Pulm**	**Neuro**
General	( ) Midline trachea	( ) No retractions	( ) AAO x 3
( ) No Acute Distress	( ) nl thyroid w/o	( ) No dullness	( ) CN II-XII intact
( ) Cooperative	enlargement	( ) No fremitus	( ) nl sensation
( ) nl Hygiene	( ) No	( ) No wheezing/	( ) Reflexes 2+ &
Eyes	lymphadenopathy	rales/rhonchi	symmetrical
( ) nl conjunctiva	**CV**	**GI**	( ) nl memory
( ) PERRLA	( ) PMI	( ) No masses/	( ) nl speech
( ) Size___	nondisplaced	tenderness	**MSK**
( ) nl Fundus	( ) No murmur/	( ) No hep/	( ) nl tone
( ) nl Discs/vessels	gallop/rub	splenomegaly	( ) nl bulk
( ) No scleral icterus	( ) nl intensity w/o	( ) nl bowel sounds	( ) nl gait
ENT	bruit	( ) No dullness	( ) nl ROM UE
( ) No scars/masses	( ) No JVD	( ) Heme (-) stool	( ) nl ROM LE
( ) nl canals/ TM	( ) nl femoral/pedal	**GU**	L___/5 UE R___/5
( ) nl hearing bilat	pulses	( ) nl ext genitalia	L___/5 LE R___/5
( ) nl teeth/tongue	( ) No pedal	( ) No hernia	
	edema		

+ PE Findings

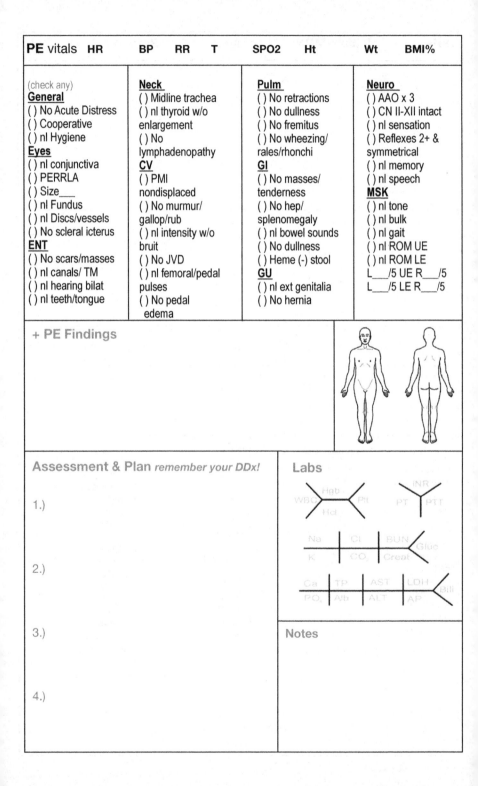

Assessment & Plan *remember your DDx!*

1.)

2.)

3.)

4.)

Labs

Notes

Date: **Initials/MRN:**   **Age:**   **Rotation:**

CC: _____ y/o M/F
HPI: *symptoms/pertinent +/- ROS/prior episodes/recent travel/sick contacts*

PMHx *child/adult illness /hospitalizations/ immunizations*	**SurgHx** *type/when/ why/complications*	**FamHx** *parents/siblings/ children*

SHx *smoker/ETOH/illicits/exercise/sex/maritalstatus*

Allergies *meds/foods/ environmental/reactions*	**Meds** *reason/dose/time/route/compliance/vitamins/ herbs/otcs*

ROS (circle any)

Gen	**Pulm**	**GU**	**Endo**
Fatigue	Cough	Dysuria	Polyuria
Weight +/-	SOB	Frequency	Polydypsia
Chills	Wheezing	Hematuria	Polyphagia
Night sweats	Hemoptysis	Discharge	**Derm**
Eyes	**CV**	Flank pain	Rash
Pain	Chest pain	**MS**	Pruritis
Redness	Edema	Arthralgia	Wound(s)
Vision changes	PND	Arthritis	**Neuro**
ENT	Orthopnea	Joint swelling	Weakness
Headache	Palpitations	Myalgias	Seizures
Hoarseness	Claudication	Back pain	Parasthesias
Sore throat	**GI**	**Heme**	Tremors
Sinus sx	Abd pain	Bleeding	Syncope
Hearing loss	N/V	Bruising	**Psych**
Tinnitus	Heartburn	**Lymph**	Anxiety
Runny nose	Bloody stools	Swelling	Depression

+ ROS Findings

PE vitals HR	BP RR T	SPO2 Ht	Wt BMI%

(check any)	**Neck**	**Pulm**	**Neuro**
General	( ) Midline trachea	( ) No retractions	( ) AAO x 3
( ) No Acute Distress	( ) nl thyroid w/o	( ) No dullness	( ) CN II-XII intact
( ) Cooperative	enlargement	( ) No fremitus	( ) nl sensation
( ) nl Hygiene	( ) No	( ) No wheezing/	( ) Reflexes 2+ &
Eyes	lymphadenopathy	rales/rhonchi	symmetrical
( ) nl conjunctiva	**CV**	**GI**	( ) nl memory
( ) PERRLA	( ) PMI	( ) No masses/	( ) nl speech
( ) Size___	nondisplaced	tenderness	**MSK**
( ) nl Fundus	( ) No murmur/	( ) No hep/	( ) nl tone
( ) nl Discs/vessels	gallop/rub	splenomegaly	( ) nl bulk
( ) No scleral icterus	( ) nl intensity w/o	( ) nl bowel sounds	( ) nl gait
ENT	bruit	( ) No dullness	( ) nl ROM UE
( ) No scars/masses	( ) No JVD	( ) Heme (-) stool	( ) nl ROM LE
( ) nl canals/ TM	( ) nl femoral/pedal	**GU**	L___/5 UE R___/5
( ) nl hearing bilat	pulses	( ) nl ext genitalia	L___/5 LE R___/5
( ) nl teeth/tongue	( ) No pedal	( ) No hernia	
	edema		

+ PE Findings

Assessment & Plan *remember your DDx!*

1.)

2.)

3.)

4.)

Labs

Notes

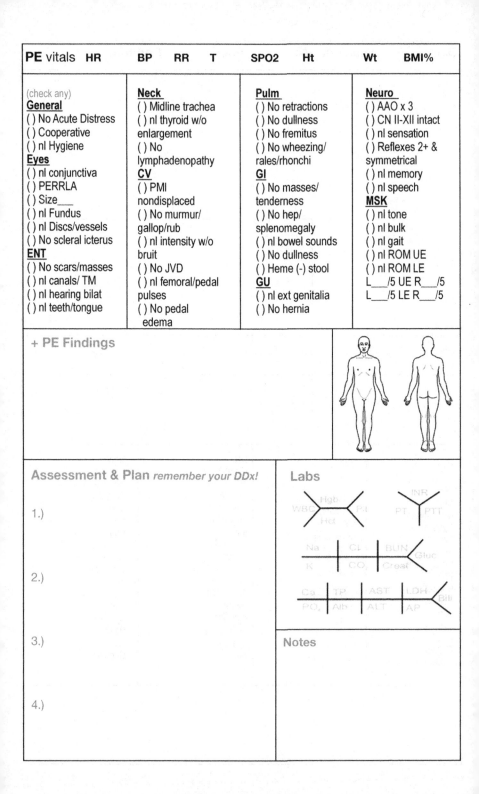

Date: **Initials/MRN:**   **Age:**   **Rotation:**

CC: _____ y/o M/F
HPI: *symptoms/pertinent +/- ROS/prior episodes/recent travel/sick contacts*

PMHx *child/adult illness /hospitalizations/ immunizations*

SurgHx *type/when/ why/complications*

FamHx *parents/siblings/ children*

SHx *smoker/ETOH/illicits/exercise/sex/maritalstatus*

Allergies *meds/foods/ environmental/reactions*

Meds *reason/dose/time/route/compliance/vitamins/ herbs/otcs*

ROS (circle any)

Gen
Fatigue
Weight +/-
Chills
Night sweats
Eyes
Pain
Redness
Vision changes
ENT
Headache
Hoarseness
Sore throat
Sinus sx
Hearing loss
Tinnitus
Runny nose

Pulm
Cough
SOB
Wheezing
Hemoptysis
CV
Chest pain
Edema
PND
Orthopnea
Palpitations
Claudication
GI
Abd pain
N/V
Heartburn
Bloody stools

GU
Dysuria
Frequency
Hematuria
Discharge
Flank pain
MS
Arthralgia
Arthritis
Joint swelling
Myalgias
Back pain
Heme
Bleeding
Bruising
Lymph
Swelling

Endo
Polyuria
Polydypsia
Polyphagia
Derm
Rash
Pruritis
Wound(s)
Neuro
Weakness
Seizures
Parasthesias
Tremors
Syncope
Psych
Anxiety
Depression

+ ROS Findings

PE vitals **HR** **BP** **RR** **T** **SPO2** **Ht** **Wt** **BMI%**

(check any)	**Neck**	**Pulm**	**Neuro**
General	( ) Midline trachea	( ) No retractions	( ) AAO x 3
( ) No Acute Distress	( ) nl thyroid w/o	( ) No dullness	( ) CN II-XII intact
( ) Cooperative	enlargement	( ) No fremitus	( ) nl sensation
( ) nl Hygiene	( ) No	( ) No wheezing/	( ) Reflexes 2+ &
Eyes	lymphadenopathy	rales/rhonchi	symmetrical
( ) nl conjunctiva	**CV**	**GI**	( ) nl memory
( ) PERRLA	( ) PMI	( ) No masses/	( ) nl speech
( ) Size___	nondisplaced	tenderness	**MSK**
( ) nl Fundus	( ) No murmur/	( ) No hep/	( ) nl tone
( ) nl Discs/vessels	gallop/rub	splenomegaly	( ) nl bulk
( ) No scleral icterus	( ) nl intensity w/o	( ) nl bowel sounds	( ) nl gait
ENT	bruit	( ) No dullness	( ) nl ROM UE
( ) No scars/masses	( ) No JVD	( ) Heme (-) stool	( ) nl ROM LE
( ) nl canals/ TM	( ) nl femoral/pedal	**GU**	L___/5 UE R___/5
( ) nl hearing bilat	pulses	( ) nl ext genitalia	L___/5 LE R___/5
( ) nl teeth/tongue	( ) No pedal	( ) No hernia	
	edema		

+ PE Findings

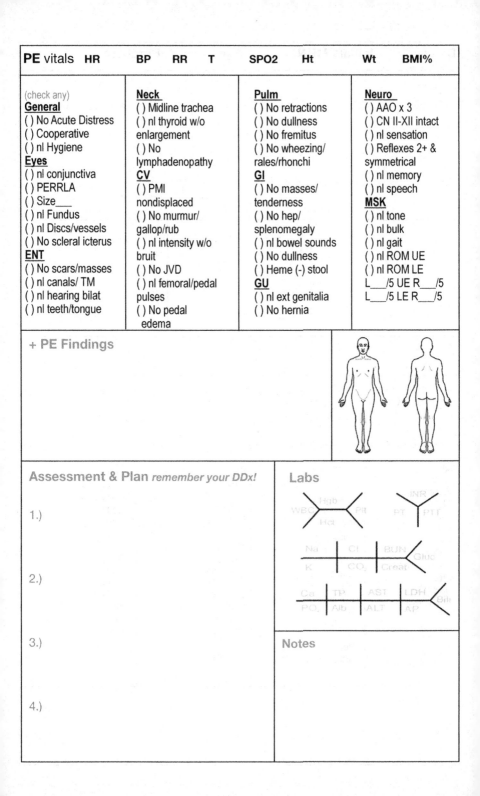

Assessment & Plan *remember your DDx!*

1.)

2.)

3.)

4.)

Labs

Hgb
WBC   Plt
Hct

INR
PT   PTT

Na   Cl   BUN
                      Gluc
K   CO₂   Creat

Ca   TP   AST   LDH
                           Bili
PO₄ Alb   ALT   AP

Notes

Date:	Initials/MRN:	Age:	Rotation:

CC: _____ y/o M/F
HPI: *symptoms/pertinent +/- ROS/prior episodes/recent travel/sick contacts*

PMHx *child/adult illness /hospitalizations/ immunizations*	**SurgHx** *type/when/ why/complications*	**FamHx** *parents/siblings/ children*

SHx *smoker/ETOH/illicits/exercise/sex/maritalstatus*

Allergies *meds/foods/ environmental/reactions*	**Meds** *reason/dose/time/route/compliance/vitamins/ herbs/otcs*

ROS (circle any)

Gen	**Pulm**	**GU**	**Endo**
Fatigue	Cough	Dysuria	Polyuria
Weight +/-	SOB	Frequency	Polydypsia
Chills	Wheezing	Hematuria	Polyphagia
Night sweats	Hemoptysis	Discharge	**Derm**
Eyes	**CV**	Flank pain	Rash
Pain	Chest pain	**MS**	Pruritis
Redness	Edema	Arthralgia	Wound(s)
Vision changes	PND	Arthritis	**Neuro**
ENT	Orthopnea	Joint swelling	Weakness
Headache	Palpitations	Myalgias	Seizures
Hoarseness	Claudication	Back pain	Parasthesias
Sore throat	**GI**	**Heme**	Tremors
Sinus sx	Abd pain	Bleeding	Syncope
Hearing loss	N/V	Bruising	**Psych**
Tinnitus	Heartburn	**Lymph**	Anxiety
Runny nose	Bloody stools	Swelling	Depression

+ ROS Findings

PE vitals	HR	BP	RR	T	SPO2	Ht	Wt	BMI%

(check any) **General** ( ) No Acute Distress ( ) Cooperative ( ) nl Hygiene **Eyes** ( ) nl conjunctiva ( ) PERRLA ( ) Size___ ( ) nl Fundus ( ) nl Discs/vessels ( ) No scleral icterus **ENT** ( ) No scars/masses ( ) nl canals/ TM ( ) nl hearing bilat ( ) nl teeth/tongue	**Neck** ( ) Midline trachea ( ) nl thyroid w/o enlargement ( ) No lymphadenopathy **CV** ( ) PMI nondisplaced ( ) No murmur/ gallop/rub ( ) nl intensity w/o bruit ( ) No JVD ( ) nl femoral/pedal pulses ( ) No pedal edema	**Pulm** ( ) No retractions ( ) No dullness ( ) No fremitus ( ) No wheezing/ rales/rhonchi **GI** ( ) No masses/ tenderness ( ) No hep/ splenomegaly ( ) nl bowel sounds ( ) No dullness ( ) Heme (-) stool **GU** ( ) nl ext genitalia ( ) No hernia	**Neuro** ( ) AAO x 3 ( ) CN II-XII intact ( ) nl sensation ( ) Reflexes 2+ & symmetrical ( ) nl memory ( ) nl speech **MSK** ( ) nl tone ( ) nl bulk ( ) nl gait ( ) nl ROM UE ( ) nl ROM LE L___/5 UE R___/5 L___/5 LE R___/5

+ PE Findings

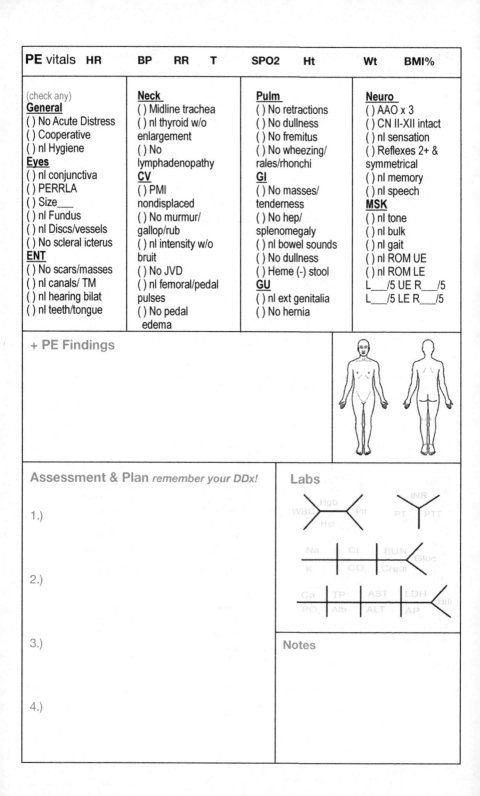

Assessment & Plan *remember your DDx!*

1.)

2.)

3.)

4.)

Labs

Hgb
WBC   Plt
Hct

INR
PT   PTT

Na   Cl   BUN
                        Gluc
K   CO₂   Creat

Ca   TP   AST   LDH
                          Bili
PO₄ Alb ALT   AP

Notes

Date:	Initials/MRN:	Age:	Rotation:

CC: _____ y/o M/F
HPI: *symptoms/pertinent +/- ROS/prior episodes/recent travel/sick contacts*

PMHx *child/adult illness /hospitalizations/ immunizations*	**SurgHx** *type/when/ why/complications*	**FamHx** *parents/siblings/ children*

SHx *smoker/ETOH/illicits/exercise/sex/maritalstatus*

Allergies *meds/foods/ environmental/reactions*	**Meds** *reason/dose/time/route/compliance/vitamins/ herbs/otcs*

ROS (circle any)

Gen	**Pulm**	**GU**	**Endo**
Fatigue	Cough	Dysuria	Polyuria
Weight +/-	SOB	Frequency	Polydypsia
Chills	Wheezing	Hematuria	Polyphagia
Night sweats	Hemoptysis	Discharge	**Derm**
Eyes	**CV**	Flank pain	Rash
Pain	Chest pain	**MS**	Pruritis
Redness	Edema	Arthralgia	Wound(s)
Vision changes	PND	Arthritis	**Neuro**
ENT	Orthopnea	Joint swelling	Weakness
Headache	Palpitations	Myalgias	Seizures
Hoarseness	Claudication	Back pain	Parasthesias
Sore throat	**GI**	**Heme**	Tremors
Sinus sx	Abd pain	Bleeding	Syncope
Hearing loss	N/V	Bruising	**Psych**
Tinnitus	Heartburn	**Lymph**	Anxiety
Runny nose	Bloody stools	Swelling	Depression

+ ROS Findings

PE vitals	**HR**	**BP**	**RR**	**T**	**SPO2**	**Ht**	**Wt**	**BMI%**

(check any)

General
( ) No Acute Distress
( ) Cooperative
( ) nl Hygiene

Eyes
( ) nl conjunctiva
( ) PERRLA
( ) Size___
( ) nl Fundus
( ) nl Discs/vessels
( ) No scleral icterus

ENT
( ) No scars/masses
( ) nl canals/ TM
( ) nl hearing bilat
( ) nl teeth/tongue

Neck
( ) Midline trachea
( ) nl thyroid w/o enlargement
( ) No lymphadenopathy

CV
( ) PMI nondisplaced
( ) No murmur/ gallop/rub
( ) nl intensity w/o bruit
( ) No JVD
( ) nl femoral/pedal pulses
( ) No pedal edema

Pulm
( ) No retractions
( ) No dullness
( ) No fremitus
( ) No wheezing/ rales/rhonchi

GI
( ) No masses/ tenderness
( ) No hep/ splenomegaly
( ) nl bowel sounds
( ) No dullness
( ) Heme (-) stool

GU
( ) nl ext genitalia
( ) No hernia

Neuro
( ) AAO x 3
( ) CN II-XII intact
( ) nl sensation
( ) Reflexes 2+ & symmetrical
( ) nl memory
( ) nl speech

MSK
( ) nl tone
( ) nl bulk
( ) nl gait
( ) nl ROM UE
( ) nl ROM LE
L___/5 UE R___/5
L___/5 LE R___/5

+ PE Findings

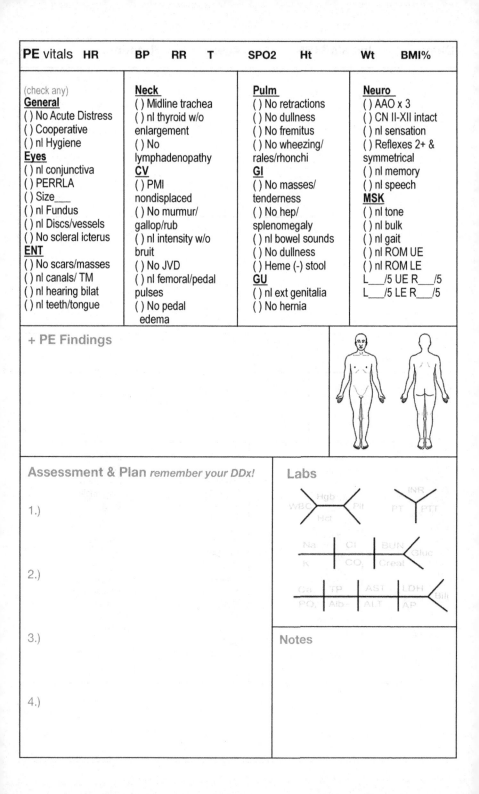

Assessment & Plan *remember your DDx!*

1.)

2.)

3.)

4.)

Labs

Notes

Date:	Initials/MRN:	Age:	Rotation:

CC: _____ y/o M/F

HPI: *symptoms/pertinent +/- ROS/prior episodes/recent travel/sick contacts*

PMHx *child/adult illness /hospitalizations/ immunizations*	**SurgHx** *type/when/ why/complications*	**FamHx** *parents/siblings/ children*

SHx *smoker/ETOH/illicits/exercise/sex/maritalstatus*

Allergies *meds/foods/ environmental/reactions*	**Meds** *reason/dose/time/route/compliance/vitamins/ herbs/otcs*

ROS (circle any)

Gen	**Pulm**	**GU**	**Endo**
Fatigue	Cough	Dysuria	Polyuria
Weight +/-	SOB	Frequency	Polydypsia
Chills	Wheezing	Hematuria	Polyphagia
Night sweats	Hemoptysis	Discharge	**Derm**
Eyes	**CV**	Flank pain	Rash
Pain	Chest pain	**MS**	Pruritis
Redness	Edema	Arthralgia	Wound(s)
Vision changes	PND	Arthritis	**Neuro**
ENT	Orthopnea	Joint swelling	Weakness
Headache	Palpitations	Myalgias	Seizures
Hoarseness	Claudication	Back pain	Parasthesias
Sore throat	**GI**	**Heme**	Tremors
Sinus sx	Abd pain	Bleeding	Syncope
Hearing loss	N/V	Bruising	**Psych**
Tinnitus	Heartburn	**Lymph**	Anxiety
Runny nose	Bloody stools	Swelling	Depression

+ ROS Findings

PE vitals	**HR**	**BP**	**RR**	**T**	**SPO2**	**Ht**	**Wt**	**BMI%**

(check any)

General
( ) No Acute Distress
( ) Cooperative
( ) nl Hygiene
Eyes
( ) nl conjunctiva
( ) PERRLA
( ) Size___
( ) nl Fundus
( ) nl Discs/vessels
( ) No scleral icterus
ENT
( ) No scars/masses
( ) nl canals/ TM
( ) nl hearing bilat
( ) nl teeth/tongue

Neck
( ) Midline trachea
( ) nl thyroid w/o
enlargement
( ) No
lymphadenopathy
CV
( ) PMI
nondisplaced
( ) No murmur/
gallop/rub
( ) nl intensity w/o
bruit
( ) No JVD
( ) nl femoral/pedal
pulses
( ) No pedal
edema

Pulm
( ) No retractions
( ) No dullness
( ) No fremitus
( ) No wheezing/
rales/rhonchi
GI
( ) No masses/
tenderness
( ) No hep/
splenomegaly
( ) nl bowel sounds
( ) No dullness
( ) Heme (-) stool
GU
( ) nl ext genitalia
( ) No hernia

Neuro
( ) AAO x 3
( ) CN II-XII intact
( ) nl sensation
( ) Reflexes 2+ &
symmetrical
( ) nl memory
( ) nl speech
MSK
( ) nl tone
( ) nl bulk
( ) nl gait
( ) nl ROM UE
( ) nl ROM LE
L___/5 UE R___/5
L___/5 LE R___/5

+ PE Findings

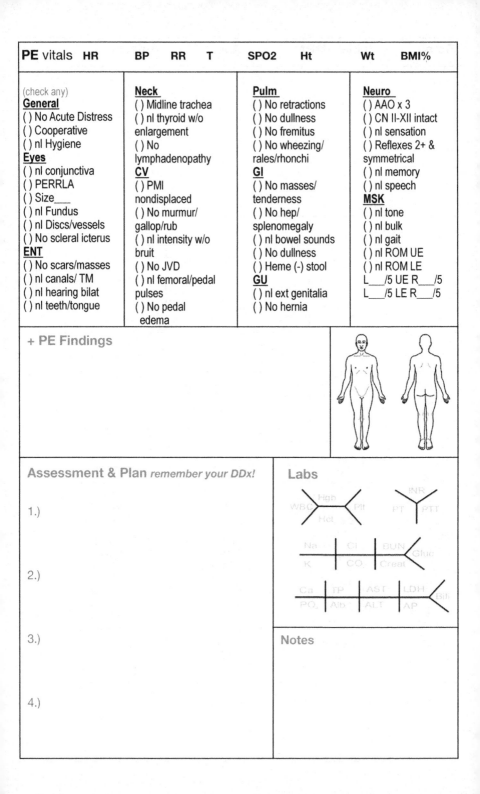

Assessment & Plan *remember your DDx!*

1.)

2.)

3.)

4.)

Labs

Notes

Date: **Initials/MRN:**   **Age:**   **Rotation:**

CC: _____ y/o M/F
HPI: *symptoms/pertinent +/- ROS/prior episodes/recent travel/sick contacts*

PMHx *child/adult illness /hospitalizations/ immunizations*	**SurgHx** *type/when/ why/complications*	**FamHx** *parents/siblings/ children*

SHx *smoker/ETOH/illicits/exercise/sex/maritalstatus*

Allergies *meds/foods/ environmental/reactions*	**Meds** *reason/dose/time/route/compliance/vitamins/ herbs/otcs*

ROS (circle any)

Gen	**Pulm**	**GU**	**Endo**
Fatigue	Cough	Dysuria	Polyuria
Weight +/-	SOB	Frequency	Polydypsia
Chills	Wheezing	Hematuria	Polyphagia
Night sweats	Hemoptysis	Discharge	**Derm**
Eyes	**CV**	Flank pain	Rash
Pain	Chest pain	**MS**	Pruritis
Redness	Edema	Arthralgia	Wound(s)
Vision changes	PND	Arthritis	**Neuro**
ENT	Orthopnea	Joint swelling	Weakness
Headache	Palpitations	Myalgias	Seizures
Hoarseness	Claudication	Back pain	Parasthesias
Sore throat	**GI**	**Heme**	Tremors
Sinus sx	Abd pain	Bleeding	Syncope
Hearing loss	N/V	Bruising	**Psych**
Tinnitus	Heartburn	**Lymph**	Anxiety
Runny nose	Bloody stools	Swelling	Depression

+ ROS Findings

PE vitals	HR	BP	RR	T	SPO2	Ht	Wt	BMI%

(check any)

General
( ) No Acute Distress
( ) Cooperative
( ) nl Hygiene

Eyes
( ) nl conjunctiva
( ) PERRLA
( ) Size___
( ) nl Fundus
( ) nl Discs/vessels
( ) No scleral icterus

ENT
( ) No scars/masses
( ) nl canals/ TM
( ) nl hearing bilat
( ) nl teeth/tongue

Neck
( ) Midline trachea
( ) nl thyroid w/o
enlargement
( ) No
lymphadenopathy

CV
( ) PMI
nondisplaced
( ) No murmur/
gallop/rub
( ) nl intensity w/o
bruit
( ) No JVD
( ) nl femoral/pedal
pulses
( ) No pedal
edema

Pulm
( ) No retractions
( ) No dullness
( ) No fremitus
( ) No wheezing/
rales/rhonchi

GI
( ) No masses/
tenderness
( ) No hep/
splenomegaly
( ) nl bowel sounds
( ) No dullness
( ) Heme (-) stool

GU
( ) nl ext genitalia
( ) No hernia

Neuro
( ) AAO x 3
( ) CN II-XII intact
( ) nl sensation
( ) Reflexes 2+ &
symmetrical
( ) nl memory
( ) nl speech

MSK
( ) nl tone
( ) nl bulk
( ) nl gait
( ) nl ROM UE
( ) nl ROM LE
L___/5 UE R___/5
L___/5 LE R___/5

+ PE Findings

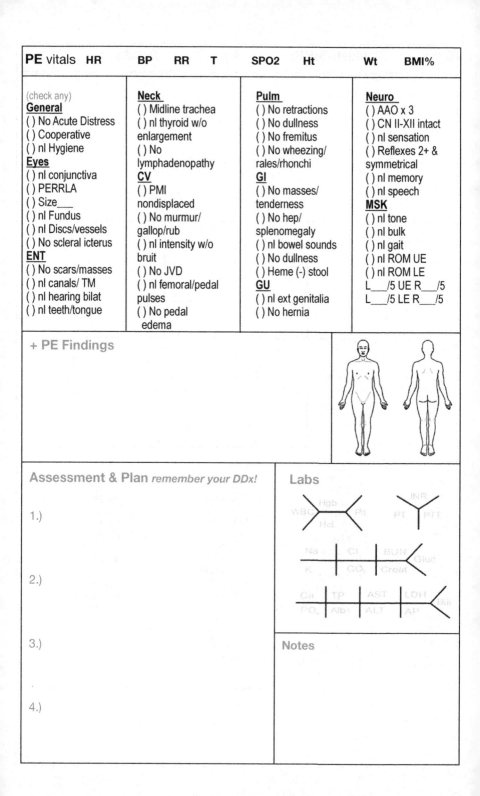

Assessment & Plan *remember your DDx!*

1.)

2.)

3.)

4.)

Labs

Notes

Date:	Initials/MRN:	Age:	Rotation:

CC: _____ y/o M/F
HPI: *symptoms/pertinent +/- ROS/prior episodes/recent travel/sick contacts*

PMHx *child/adult illness /hospitalizations/ immunizations*	**SurgHx** *type/when/ why/complications*	**FamHx** *parents/siblings/ children*

SHx *smoker/ETOH/illicits/exercise/sex/maritalstatus*

Allergies *meds/foods/ environmental/reactions*	**Meds** *reason/dose/time/route/compliance/vitamins/ herbs/otcs*

ROS (circle any)

Gen	**Pulm**	**GU**	**Endo**
Fatigue	Cough	Dysuria	Polyuria
Weight +/-	SOB	Frequency	Polydypsia
Chills	Wheezing	Hematuria	Polyphagia
Night sweats	Hemoptysis	Discharge	**Derm**
Eyes	**CV**	Flank pain	Rash
Pain	Chest pain	**MS**	Pruritis
Redness	Edema	Arthralgia	Wound(s)
Vision changes	PND	Arthritis	**Neuro**
ENT	Orthopnea	Joint swelling	Weakness
Headache	Palpitations	Myalgias	Seizures
Hoarseness	Claudication	Back pain	Parasthesias
Sore throat	**GI**	**Heme**	Tremors
Sinus sx	Abd pain	Bleeding	Syncope
Hearing loss	N/V	Bruising	**Psych**
Tinnitus	Heartburn	**Lymph**	Anxiety
Runny nose	Bloody stools	Swelling	Depression

+ ROS Findings

PE vitals	HR	BP	RR	T	SPO2	Ht	Wt	BMI%

(check any)	**Neck**	**Pulm**	**Neuro**
General	( ) Midline trachea	( ) No retractions	( ) AAO x 3
( ) No Acute Distress	( ) nl thyroid w/o	( ) No dullness	( ) CN II-XII intact
( ) Cooperative	enlargement	( ) No fremitus	( ) nl sensation
( ) nl Hygiene	( ) No	( ) No wheezing/	( ) Reflexes 2+ &
Eyes	lymphadenopathy	rales/rhonchi	symmetrical
( ) nl conjunctiva	**CV**	**GI**	( ) nl memory
( ) PERRLA	( ) PMI	( ) No masses/	( ) nl speech
( ) Size___	nondisplaced	tenderness	**MSK**
( ) nl Fundus	( ) No murmur/	( ) No hep/	( ) nl tone
( ) nl Discs/vessels	gallop/rub	splenomegaly	( ) nl bulk
( ) No scleral icterus	( ) nl intensity w/o	( ) nl bowel sounds	( ) nl gait
ENT	bruit	( ) No dullness	( ) nl ROM UE
( ) No scars/masses	( ) No JVD	( ) Heme (-) stool	( ) nl ROM LE
( ) nl canals/ TM	( ) nl femoral/pedal	**GU**	L___/5 UE R___/5
( ) nl hearing bilat	pulses	( ) nl ext genitalia	L___/5 LE R___/5
( ) nl teeth/tongue	( ) No pedal	( ) No hernia	
	edema		

+ PE Findings

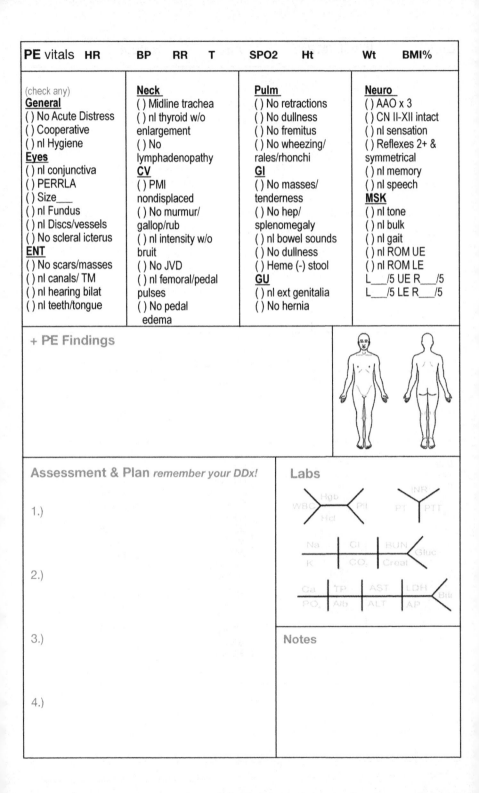

Assessment & Plan *remember your DDx!*

1.)

2.)

3.)

4.)

Labs

Notes

Date:	Initials/MRN:	Age:	Rotation:

CC: _____ y/o M/F
HPI: *symptoms/pertinent +/- ROS/prior episodes/recent travel/sick contacts*

PMHx *child/adult illness /hospitalizations/ immunizations*	**SurgHx** *type/when/ why/complications*	**FamHx** *parents/siblings/ children*

SHx *smoker/ETOH/illicits/exercise/sex/maritalstatus*

Allergies *meds/foods/ environmental/reactions*	**Meds** *reason/dose/time/route/compliance/vitamins/ herbs/otcs*

ROS (circle any)

Gen	**Pulm**	**GU**	**Endo**
Fatigue	Cough	Dysuria	Polyuria
Weight +/-	SOB	Frequency	Polydypsia
Chills	Wheezing	Hematuria	Polyphagia
Night sweats	Hemoptysis	Discharge	**Derm**
Eyes	**CV**	Flank pain	Rash
Pain	Chest pain	**MS**	Pruritis
Redness	Edema	Arthralgia	Wound(s)
Vision changes	PND	Arthritis	**Neuro**
ENT	Orthopnea	Joint swelling	Weakness
Headache	Palpitations	Myalgias	Seizures
Hoarseness	Claudication	Back pain	Parasthesias
Sore throat	**GI**	**Heme**	Tremors
Sinus sx	Abd pain	Bleeding	Syncope
Hearing loss	N/V	Bruising	**Psych**
Tinnitus	Heartburn	**Lymph**	Anxiety
Runny nose	Bloody stools	Swelling	Depression

+ ROS Findings

PE vitals **HR**   **BP**   **RR**   **T**   **SPO2**   **Ht**   **Wt**   **BMI%**

(check any)	**Neck**	**Pulm**	**Neuro**
General	( ) Midline trachea	( ) No retractions	( ) AAO x 3
( ) No Acute Distress	( ) nl thyroid w/o	( ) No dullness	( ) CN II-XII intact
( ) Cooperative	enlargement	( ) No fremitus	( ) nl sensation
( ) nl Hygiene	( ) No	( ) No wheezing/	( ) Reflexes 2+ &
Eyes	lymphadenopathy	rales/rhonchi	symmetrical
( ) nl conjunctiva	**CV**	**GI**	( ) nl memory
( ) PERRLA	( ) PMI	( ) No masses/	( ) nl speech
( ) Size___	nondisplaced	tenderness	**MSK**
( ) nl Fundus	( ) No murmur/	( ) No hep/	( ) nl tone
( ) nl Discs/vessels	gallop/rub	splenomegaly	( ) nl bulk
( ) No scleral icterus	( ) nl intensity w/o	( ) nl bowel sounds	( ) nl gait
ENT	bruit	( ) No dullness	( ) nl ROM UE
( ) No scars/masses	( ) No JVD	( ) Heme (-) stool	( ) nl ROM LE
( ) nl canals/ TM	( ) nl femoral/pedal	**GU**	L___/5 UE R___/5
( ) nl hearing bilat	pulses	( ) nl ext genitalia	L___/5 LE R___/5
( ) nl teeth/tongue	( ) No pedal	( ) No hernia	
	edema		

+ PE Findings

Assessment & Plan *remember your DDx!*

1.)

2.)

3.)

4.)

Labs

Notes

Date:	Initials/MRN:	Age:	Rotation:

CC: _____ y/o M/F
HPI: *symptoms/pertinent +/- ROS/prior episodes/recent travel/sick contacts*

PMHx *child/adult illness /hospitalizations/ immunizations*	**SurgHx** *type/when/ why/complications*	**FamHx** *parents/siblings/ children*

SHx *smoker/ETOH/illicits/exercise/sex/maritalstatus*

Allergies *meds/foods/ environmental/reactions*	**Meds** *reason/dose/time/route/compliance/vitamins/ herbs/otcs*

ROS (circle any)

Gen	**Pulm**	**GU**	**Endo**
Fatigue	Cough	Dysuria	Polyuria
Weight +/-	SOB	Frequency	Polydypsia
Chills	Wheezing	Hematuria	Polyphagia
Night sweats	Hemoptysis	Discharge	**Derm**
Eyes	**CV**	Flank pain	Rash
Pain	Chest pain	**MS**	Pruritis
Redness	Edema	Arthralgia	Wound(s)
Vision changes	PND	Arthritis	**Neuro**
ENT	Orthopnea	Joint swelling	Weakness
Headache	Palpitations	Myalgias	Seizures
Hoarseness	Claudication	Back pain	Parasthesias
Sore throat	**GI**	**Heme**	Tremors
Sinus sx	Abd pain	Bleeding	Syncope
Hearing loss	N/V	Bruising	**Psych**
Tinnitus	Heartburn	**Lymph**	Anxiety
Runny nose	Bloody stools	Swelling	Depression

+ ROS Findings

PE vitals **HR**   **BP**   **RR**   **T**   **SPO2**   **Ht**   **Wt**   **BMI%**

(check any)	**Neck**	**Pulm**	**Neuro**
General	( ) Midline trachea	( ) No retractions	( ) AAO x 3
( ) No Acute Distress	( ) nl thyroid w/o	( ) No dullness	( ) CN II-XII intact
( ) Cooperative	enlargement	( ) No fremitus	( ) nl sensation
( ) nl Hygiene	( ) No	( ) No wheezing/	( ) Reflexes 2+ &
Eyes	lymphadenopathy	rales/rhonchi	symmetrical
( ) nl conjunctiva	**CV**	**GI**	( ) nl memory
( ) PERRLA	( ) PMI	( ) No masses/	( ) nl speech
( ) Size___	nondisplaced	tenderness	**MSK**
( ) nl Fundus	( ) No murmur/	( ) No hep/	( ) nl tone
( ) nl Discs/vessels	gallop/rub	splenomegaly	( ) nl bulk
( ) No scleral icterus	( ) nl intensity w/o	( ) nl bowel sounds	( ) nl gait
ENT	bruit	( ) No dullness	( ) nl ROM UE
( ) No scars/masses	( ) No JVD	( ) Heme (-) stool	( ) nl ROM LE
( ) nl canals/ TM	( ) nl femoral/pedal	**GU**	L___/5 UE R___/5
( ) nl hearing bilat	pulses	( ) nl ext genitalia	L___/5 LE R___/5
( ) nl teeth/tongue	( ) No pedal	( ) No hernia	
	edema		

+ PE Findings

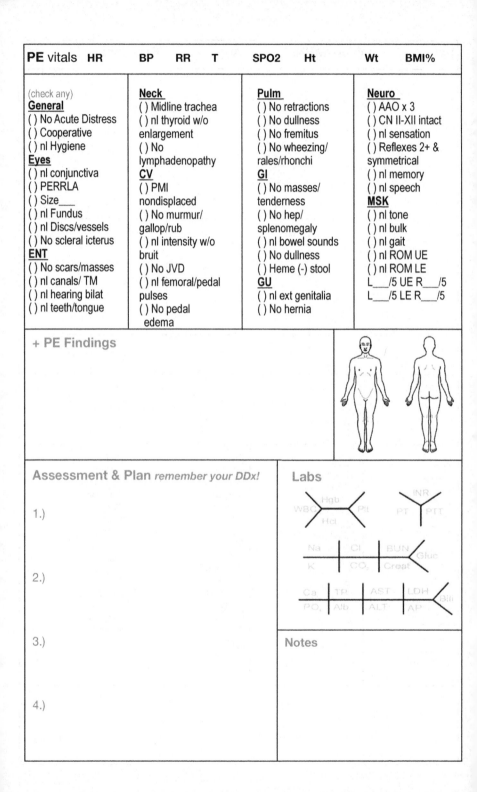

Assessment & Plan *remember your DDx!*

1.)

2.)

3.)

4.)

Labs

Notes

Date:	Initials/MRN:	Age:	Rotation:

CC: _____ y/o M/F
HPI: *symptoms/pertinent +/- ROS/prior episodes/recent travel/sick contacts*

PMHx *child/adult illness /hospitalizations/ immunizations*	**SurgHx** *type/when/ why/complications*	**FamHx** *parents/siblings/ children*

SHx *smoker/ETOH/illicits/exercise/sex/maritalstatus*

Allergies *meds/foods/ environmental/reactions*	**Meds** *reason/dose/time/route/compliance/vitamins/ herbs/otcs*

ROS (circle any)

Gen	**Pulm**	**GU**	**Endo**
Fatigue	Cough	Dysuria	Polyuria
Weight +/-	SOB	Frequency	Polydypsia
Chills	Wheezing	Hematuria	Polyphagia
Night sweats	Hemoptysis	Discharge	**Derm**
Eyes	**CV**	Flank pain	Rash
Pain	Chest pain	**MS**	Pruritis
Redness	Edema	Arthralgia	Wound(s)
Vision changes	PND	Arthritis	**Neuro**
ENT	Orthopnea	Joint swelling	Weakness
Headache	Palpitations	Myalgias	Seizures
Hoarseness	Claudication	Back pain	Parasthesias
Sore throat	**GI**	**Heme**	Tremors
Sinus sx	Abd pain	Bleeding	Syncope
Hearing loss	N/V	Bruising	**Psych**
Tinnitus	Heartburn	**Lymph**	Anxiety
Runny nose	Bloody stools	Swelling	Depression

+ ROS Findings

PE vitals	**HR**	**BP**	**RR**	**T**	**SPO2**	**Ht**	**Wt**	**BMI%**

(check any)

General
( ) No Acute Distress
( ) Cooperative
( ) nl Hygiene
Eyes
( ) nl conjunctiva
( ) PERRLA
( ) Size___
( ) nl Fundus
( ) nl Discs/vessels
( ) No scleral icterus
ENT
( ) No scars/masses
( ) nl canals/ TM
( ) nl hearing bilat
( ) nl teeth/tongue

Neck
( ) Midline trachea
( ) nl thyroid w/o enlargement
( ) No lymphadenopathy
CV
( ) PMI nondisplaced
( ) No murmur/ gallop/rub
( ) nl intensity w/o bruit
( ) No JVD
( ) nl femoral/pedal pulses
( ) No pedal edema

Pulm
( ) No retractions
( ) No dullness
( ) No fremitus
( ) No wheezing/ rales/rhonchi
GI
( ) No masses/ tenderness
( ) No hep/ splenomegaly
( ) nl bowel sounds
( ) No dullness
( ) Heme (-) stool
GU
( ) nl ext genitalia
( ) No hernia

Neuro
( ) AAO x 3
( ) CN II-XII intact
( ) nl sensation
( ) Reflexes 2+ & symmetrical
( ) nl memory
( ) nl speech
MSK
( ) nl tone
( ) nl bulk
( ) nl gait
( ) nl ROM UE
( ) nl ROM LE
L___/5 UE R___/5
L___/5 LE R___/5

+ PE Findings

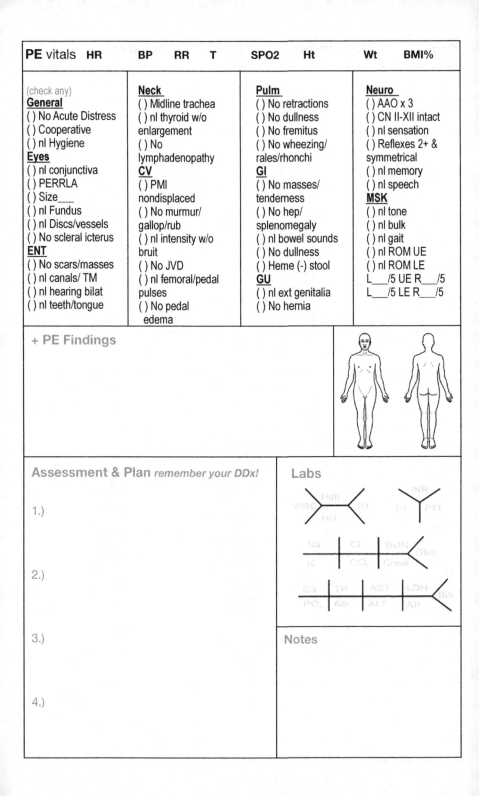

Assessment & Plan *remember your DDx!*

1.)

2.)

3.)

4.)

Labs

Notes

Date:	Initials/MRN:	Age:	Rotation:

CC: _____ y/o M/F
HPI: *symptoms/pertinent +/- ROS/prior episodes/recent travel/sick contacts*

PMHx *child/adult illness /hospitalizations/ immunizations*	**SurgHx** *type/when/ why/complications*	**FamHx** *parents/siblings/ children*

SHx *smoker/ETOH/illicits/exercise/sex/maritalstatus*

Allergies *meds/foods/ environmental/reactions*	**Meds** *reason/dose/time/route/compliance/vitamins/ herbs/otcs*

ROS (circle any)

Gen	**Pulm**	**GU**	**Endo**
Fatigue	Cough	Dysuria	Polyuria
Weight +/-	SOB	Frequency	Polydypsia
Chills	Wheezing	Hematuria	Polyphagia
Night sweats	Hemoptysis	Discharge	**Derm**
Eyes	**CV**	Flank pain	Rash
Pain	Chest pain	**MS**	Pruritis
Redness	Edema	Arthralgia	Wound(s)
Vision changes	PND	Arthritis	**Neuro**
ENT	Orthopnea	Joint swelling	Weakness
Headache	Palpitations	Myalgias	Seizures
Hoarseness	Claudication	Back pain	Parasthesias
Sore throat	**GI**	**Heme**	Tremors
Sinus sx	Abd pain	Bleeding	Syncope
Hearing loss	N/V	Bruising	**Psych**
Tinnitus	Heartburn	**Lymph**	Anxiety
Runny nose	Bloody stools	Swelling	Depression

+ ROS Findings

PE vitals	HR	BP	RR	T	SPO2	Ht	Wt	BMI%

(check any)	**Neck**	**Pulm**	**Neuro**
General	( ) Midline trachea	( ) No retractions	( ) AAO x 3
( ) No Acute Distress	( ) nl thyroid w/o	( ) No dullness	( ) CN II-XII intact
( ) Cooperative	enlargement	( ) No fremitus	( ) nl sensation
( ) nl Hygiene	( ) No	( ) No wheezing/	( ) Reflexes 2+ &
Eyes	lymphadenopathy	rales/rhonchi	symmetrical
( ) nl conjunctiva	**CV**	**GI**	( ) nl memory
( ) PERRLA	( ) PMI	( ) No masses/	( ) nl speech
( ) Size___	nondisplaced	tenderness	**MSK**
( ) nl Fundus	( ) No murmur/	( ) No hep/	( ) nl tone
( ) nl Discs/vessels	gallop/rub	splenomegaly	( ) nl bulk
( ) No scleral icterus	( ) nl intensity w/o	( ) nl bowel sounds	( ) nl gait
ENT	bruit	( ) No dullness	( ) nl ROM UE
( ) No scars/masses	( ) No JVD	( ) Heme (-) stool	( ) nl ROM LE
( ) nl canals/ TM	( ) nl femoral/pedal	**GU**	L___/5 UE R___/5
( ) nl hearing bilat	pulses	( ) nl ext genitalia	L___/5 LE R___/5
( ) nl teeth/tongue	( ) No pedal	( ) No hernia	
	edema		

+ PE Findings

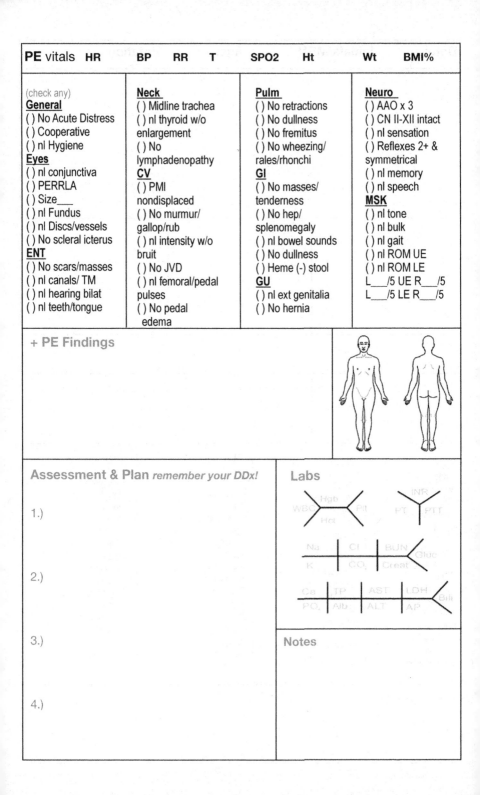

Assessment & Plan *remember your DDx!*

1.)

2.)

3.)

4.)

Labs

Hgb
WBC — Plt   INR
Hct   PT — PTT

Na | Cl | BUN
                Gluc
K | CO₂ | Creat

Ca | TP | AST | LDH
                Bili
PO₄ | Alb | ALT | AP

Notes

Date: **Initials/MRN:**   **Age:**   **Rotation:**

CC: _____ y/o M/F
HPI: *symptoms/pertinent +/- ROS/prior episodes/recent travel/sick contacts*

PMHx *child/adult illness /hospitalizations/ immunizations*	**SurgHx** *type/when/ why/complications*	**FamHx** *parents/siblings/ children*

SHx *smoker/ETOH/illicits/exercise/sex/maritalstatus*

Allergies *meds/foods/ environmental/reactions*	**Meds** *reason/dose/time/route/compliance/vitamins/ herbs/otcs*

ROS (circle any)

Gen Fatigue Weight +/- Chills Night sweats **Eyes** Pain Redness Vision changes **ENT** Headache Hoarseness Sore throat Sinus sx Hearing loss Tinnitus Runny nose	**Pulm** Cough SOB Wheezing Hemoptysis **CV** Chest pain Edema PND Orthopnea Palpitations Claudication **GI** Abd pain N/V Heartburn Bloody stools	**GU** Dysuria Frequency Hematuria Discharge Flank pain **MS** Arthralgia Arthritis Joint swelling Myalgias Back pain **Heme** Bleeding Bruising **Lymph** Swelling	**Endo** Polyuria Polydypsia Polyphagia **Derm** Rash Pruritis Wound(s) **Neuro** Weakness Seizures Parasthesias Tremors Syncope **Psych** Anxiety Depression

+ ROS Findings

PE vitals   **HR**   **BP**   **RR**   **T**   **SPO2**   **Ht**   **Wt**   **BMI%**

(check any) **General**	**Neck**	**Pulm**	**Neuro**
( ) No Acute Distress	( ) Midline trachea	( ) No retractions	( ) AAO x 3
( ) Cooperative	( ) nl thyroid w/o	( ) No dullness	( ) CN II-XII intact
( ) nl Hygiene	enlargement	( ) No fremitus	( ) nl sensation
Eyes	( ) No	( ) No wheezing/	( ) Reflexes 2+ &
( ) nl conjunctiva	lymphadenopathy	rales/rhonchi	symmetrical
( ) PERRLA	**CV**	**GI**	( ) nl memory
( ) Size___	( ) PMI	( ) No masses/	( ) nl speech
( ) nl Fundus	nondisplaced	tenderness	**MSK**
( ) nl Discs/vessels	( ) No murmur/	( ) No hep/	( ) nl tone
( ) No scleral icterus	gallop/rub	splenomegaly	( ) nl bulk
ENT	( ) nl intensity w/o	( ) nl bowel sounds	( ) nl gait
( ) No scars/masses	bruit	( ) No dullness	( ) nl ROM UE
( ) nl canals/ TM	( ) No JVD	( ) Heme (-) stool	( ) nl ROM LE
( ) nl hearing bilat	( ) nl femoral/pedal	**GU**	L___/5 UE R___/5
( ) nl teeth/tongue	pulses	( ) nl ext genitalia	L___/5 LE R___/5
	( ) No pedal	( ) No hernia	
	edema		

+ PE Findings

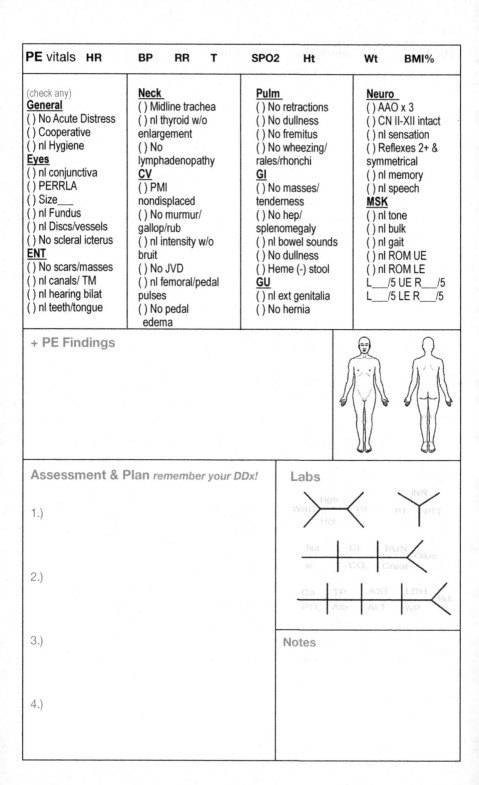

Assessment & Plan *remember your DDx!*

1.)

2.)

3.)

4.)

Labs

WBC Hgb Plt
Hct

INR
PT PTT

Na Cl BUN
K CO₂ Creat Gluc

Ca TP AST LDH
PO₄ Alb ALT AP Bili

Notes

Date:	Initials/MRN:	Age:	Rotation:

CC: _____ y/o M/F
HPI: *symptoms/pertinent +/- ROS/prior episodes/recent travel/sick contacts*

PMHx *child/adult illness /hospitalizations/ immunizations*	**SurgHx** *type/when/ why/complications*	**FamHx** *parents/siblings/ children*

SHx *smoker/ETOH/illicits/exercise/sex/maritalstatus*

Allergies *meds/foods/ environmental/reactions*	**Meds** *reason/dose/time/route/compliance/vitamins/ herbs/otcs*

ROS (circle any)

Gen	**Pulm**	**GU**	**Endo**
Fatigue	Cough	Dysuria	Polyuria
Weight +/-	SOB	Frequency	Polydypsia
Chills	Wheezing	Hematuria	Polyphagia
Night sweats	Hemoptysis	Discharge	**Derm**
Eyes	**CV**	Flank pain	Rash
Pain	Chest pain	**MS**	Pruritis
Redness	Edema	Arthralgia	Wound(s)
Vision changes	PND	Arthritis	**Neuro**
ENT	Orthopnea	Joint swelling	Weakness
Headache	Palpitations	Myalgias	Seizures
Hoarseness	Claudication	Back pain	Parasthesias
Sore throat	**GI**	**Heme**	Tremors
Sinus sx	Abd pain	Bleeding	Syncope
Hearing loss	N/V	Bruising	**Psych**
Tinnitus	Heartburn	**Lymph**	Anxiety
Runny nose	Bloody stools	Swelling	Depression

+ ROS Findings

PE vitals	HR	BP	RR	T	SPO2	Ht	Wt	BMI%

(check any)	**Neck**	**Pulm**	**Neuro**
General	( ) Midline trachea	( ) No retractions	( ) AAO x 3
( ) No Acute Distress	( ) nl thyroid w/o	( ) No dullness	( ) CN II-XII intact
( ) Cooperative	enlargement	( ) No fremitus	( ) nl sensation
( ) nl Hygiene	( ) No	( ) No wheezing/	( ) Reflexes 2+ &
Eyes	lymphadenopathy	rales/rhonchi	symmetrical
( ) nl conjunctiva	**CV**	**GI**	( ) nl memory
( ) PERRLA	( ) PMI	( ) No masses/	( ) nl speech
( ) Size___	nondisplaced	tenderness	**MSK**
( ) nl Fundus	( ) No murmur/	( ) No hep/	( ) nl tone
( ) nl Discs/vessels	gallop/rub	splenomegaly	( ) nl bulk
( ) No scleral icterus	( ) nl intensity w/o	( ) nl bowel sounds	( ) nl gait
ENT	bruit	( ) No dullness	( ) nl ROM UE
( ) No scars/masses	( ) No JVD	( ) Heme (-) stool	( ) nl ROM LE
( ) nl canals/ TM	( ) nl femoral/pedal	**GU**	L___/5 UE R___/5
( ) nl hearing bilat	pulses	( ) nl ext genitalia	L___/5 LE R___/5
( ) nl teeth/tongue	( ) No pedal	( ) No hernia	
	edema		

+ PE Findings

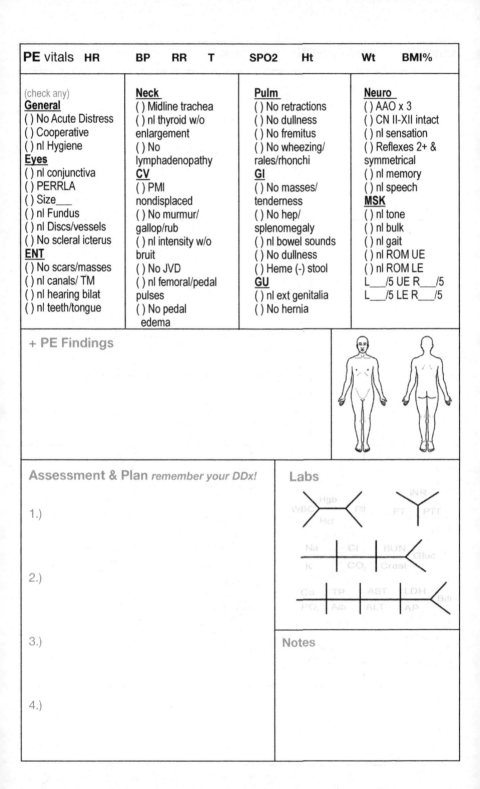

Assessment & Plan *remember your DDx!*

1.)

2.)

3.)

4.)

Labs

Notes

Date:	Initials/MRN:	Age:	Rotation:

CC: _____ y/o M/F
HPI: *symptoms/pertinent +/- ROS/prior episodes/recent travel/sick contacts*

PMHx *child/adult illness /hospitalizations/ immunizations*	**SurgHx** *type/when/ why/complications*	**FamHx** *parents/siblings/ children*

SHx *smoker/ETOH/illicits/exercise/sex/maritalstatus*

Allergies *meds/foods/ environmental/reactions*	**Meds** *reason/dose/time/route/compliance/vitamins/ herbs/otcs*

ROS (circle any)

Gen	**Pulm**	**GU**	**Endo**
Fatigue	Cough	Dysuria	Polyuria
Weight +/-	SOB	Frequency	Polydypsia
Chills	Wheezing	Hematuria	Polyphagia
Night sweats	Hemoptysis	Discharge	**Derm**
Eyes	**CV**	Flank pain	Rash
Pain	Chest pain	**MS**	Pruritis
Redness	Edema	Arthralgia	Wound(s)
Vision changes	PND	Arthritis	**Neuro**
ENT	Orthopnea	Joint swelling	Weakness
Headache	Palpitations	Myalgias	Seizures
Hoarseness	Claudication	Back pain	Parasthesias
Sore throat	**GI**	**Heme**	Tremors
Sinus sx	Abd pain	Bleeding	Syncope
Hearing loss	N/V	Bruising	**Psych**
Tinnitus	Heartburn	**Lymph**	Anxiety
Runny nose	Bloody stools	Swelling	Depression

+ ROS Findings

PE vitals	HR	BP	RR	T	SPO2	Ht	Wt	BMI%

(check any)	**Neck**	**Pulm**	**Neuro**
General	( ) Midline trachea	( ) No retractions	( ) AAO x 3
( ) No Acute Distress	( ) nl thyroid w/o	( ) No dullness	( ) CN II-XII intact
( ) Cooperative	enlargement	( ) No fremitus	( ) nl sensation
( ) nl Hygiene	( ) No	( ) No wheezing/	( ) Reflexes 2+ &
Eyes	lymphadenopathy	rales/rhonchi	symmetrical
( ) nl conjunctiva	**CV**	**GI**	( ) nl memory
( ) PERRLA	( ) PMI	( ) No masses/	( ) nl speech
( ) Size___	nondisplaced	tenderness	**MSK**
( ) nl Fundus	( ) No murmur/	( ) No hep/	( ) nl tone
( ) nl Discs/vessels	gallop/rub	splenomegaly	( ) nl bulk
( ) No scleral icterus	( ) nl intensity w/o	( ) nl bowel sounds	( ) nl gait
ENT	bruit	( ) No dullness	( ) nl ROM UE
( ) No scars/masses	( ) No JVD	( ) Heme (-) stool	( ) nl ROM LE
( ) nl canals/ TM	( ) nl femoral/pedal	**GU**	L___/5 UE R___/5
( ) nl hearing bilat	pulses	( ) nl ext genitalia	L___/5 LE R___/5
( ) nl teeth/tongue	( ) No pedal	( ) No hernia	
	edema		

+ PE Findings

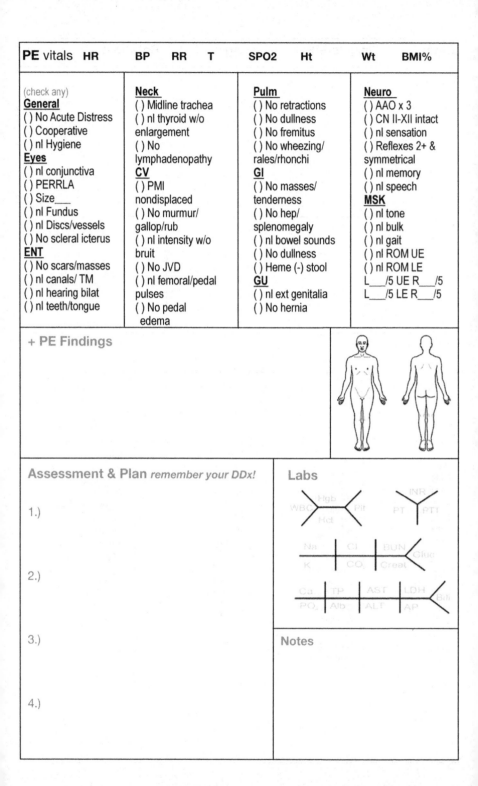

Assessment & Plan *remember your DDx!*

1.)

2.)

3.)

4.)

Labs

Hgb
WBC / Plt
Hct

INR
PT / PTT

Na | Cl | BUN
K | CO₂ | Creat | Gluc

Ca | TP | AST | LDH
PO₄ | Alb | ALT | AP | Bili

Notes

Date:	Initials/MRN:	Age:	Rotation:

CC: _____ y/o M/F
HPI: *symptoms/pertinent +/- ROS/prior episodes/recent travel/sick contacts*

PMHx *child/adult illness /hospitalizations/ immunizations*	**SurgHx** *type/when/ why/complications*	**FamHx** *parents/siblings/ children*

SHx *smoker/ETOH/illicits/exercise/sex/maritalstatus*

Allergies *meds/foods/ environmental/reactions*	**Meds** *reason/dose/time/route/compliance/vitamins/ herbs/otcs*

ROS (circle any)

Gen	**Pulm**	**GU**	**Endo**
Fatigue	Cough	Dysuria	Polyuria
Weight +/-	SOB	Frequency	Polydypsia
Chills	Wheezing	Hematuria	Polyphagia
Night sweats	Hemoptysis	Discharge	**Derm**
Eyes	**CV**	Flank pain	Rash
Pain	Chest pain	**MS**	Pruritis
Redness	Edema	Arthralgia	Wound(s)
Vision changes	PND	Arthritis	**Neuro**
ENT	Orthopnea	Joint swelling	Weakness
Headache	Palpitations	Myalgias	Seizures
Hoarseness	Claudication	Back pain	Parasthesias
Sore throat	**GI**	**Heme**	Tremors
Sinus sx	Abd pain	Bleeding	Syncope
Hearing loss	N/V	Bruising	**Psych**
Tinnitus	Heartburn	**Lymph**	Anxiety
Runny nose	Bloody stools	Swelling	Depression

+ ROS Findings

PE vitals	**HR**	**BP**	**RR**	**T**	**SPO2**	**Ht**	**Wt**	**BMI%**

(check any) **General** ( ) No Acute Distress ( ) Cooperative ( ) nl Hygiene **Eyes** ( ) nl conjunctiva ( ) PERRLA ( ) Size___ ( ) nl Fundus ( ) nl Discs/vessels ( ) No scleral icterus **ENT** ( ) No scars/masses ( ) nl canals/ TM ( ) nl hearing bilat ( ) nl teeth/tongue	**Neck** ( ) Midline trachea ( ) nl thyroid w/o enlargement ( ) No lymphadenopathy **CV** ( ) PMI nondisplaced ( ) No murmur/ gallop/rub ( ) nl intensity w/o bruit ( ) No JVD ( ) nl femoral/pedal pulses ( ) No pedal edema	**Pulm** ( ) No retractions ( ) No dullness ( ) No fremitus ( ) No wheezing/ rales/rhonchi **GI** ( ) No masses/ tenderness ( ) No hep/ splenomegaly ( ) nl bowel sounds ( ) No dullness ( ) Heme (-) stool **GU** ( ) nl ext genitalia ( ) No hernia	**Neuro** ( ) AAO x 3 ( ) CN II-XII intact ( ) nl sensation ( ) Reflexes 2+ & symmetrical ( ) nl memory ( ) nl speech **MSK** ( ) nl tone ( ) nl bulk ( ) nl gait ( ) nl ROM UE ( ) nl ROM LE L___/5 UE R___/5 L___/5 LE R___/5

+ PE Findings

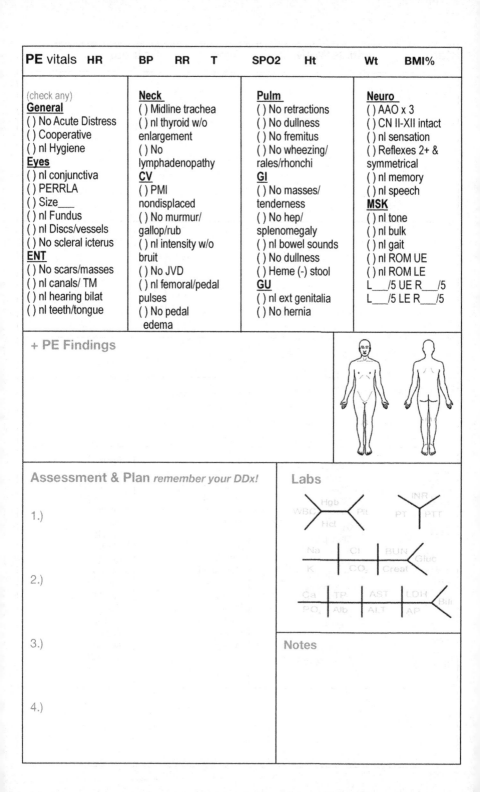

Assessment & Plan *remember your DDx!*

1.)

2.)

3.)

4.)

Labs

Notes

Date:	Initials/MRN:	Age:	Rotation:

CC: _____ y/o M/F
HPI: *symptoms/pertinent +/- ROS/prior episodes/recent travel/sick contacts*

PMHx *child/adult illness /hospitalizations/ immunizations*

SurgHx *type/when/ why/complications*

FamHx *parents/siblings/ children*

SHx *smoker/ETOH/illicits/exercise/sex/maritalstatus*

Allergies *meds/foods/ environmental/reactions*

Meds *reason/dose/time/route/compliance/vitamins/ herbs/otcs*

ROS (circle any)

Gen
Fatigue
Weight +/-
Chills
Night sweats
Eyes
Pain
Redness
Vision changes
ENT
Headache
Hoarseness
Sore throat
Sinus sx
Hearing loss
Tinnitus
Runny nose

Pulm
Cough
SOB
Wheezing
Hemoptysis
CV
Chest pain
Edema
PND
Orthopnea
Palpitations
Claudication
GI
Abd pain
N/V
Heartburn
Bloody stools

GU
Dysuria
Frequency
Hematuria
Discharge
Flank pain
MS
Arthralgia
Arthritis
Joint swelling
Myalgias
Back pain
Heme
Bleeding
Bruising
Lymph
Swelling

Endo
Polyuria
Polydypsia
Polyphagia
Derm
Rash
Pruritis
Wound(s)
Neuro
Weakness
Seizures
Parasthesias
Tremors
Syncope
Psych
Anxiety
Depression

+ ROS Findings

PE vitals	HR	BP	RR	T	SPO2	Ht	Wt	BMI%

(check any)

General
( ) No Acute Distress
( ) Cooperative
( ) nl Hygiene
Eyes
( ) nl conjunctiva
( ) PERRLA
( ) Size___
( ) nl Fundus
( ) nl Discs/vessels
( ) No scleral icterus
ENT
( ) No scars/masses
( ) nl canals/ TM
( ) nl hearing bilat
( ) nl teeth/tongue

Neck
( ) Midline trachea
( ) nl thyroid w/o enlargement
( ) No lymphadenopathy
CV
( ) PMI nondisplaced
( ) No murmur/ gallop/rub
( ) nl intensity w/o bruit
( ) No JVD
( ) nl femoral/pedal pulses
( ) No pedal edema

Pulm
( ) No retractions
( ) No dullness
( ) No fremitus
( ) No wheezing/ rales/rhonchi
GI
( ) No masses/ tenderness
( ) No hep/ splenomegaly
( ) nl bowel sounds
( ) No dullness
( ) Heme (-) stool
GU
( ) nl ext genitalia
( ) No hernia

Neuro
( ) AAO x 3
( ) CN II-XII intact
( ) nl sensation
( ) Reflexes 2+ & symmetrical
( ) nl memory
( ) nl speech
MSK
( ) nl tone
( ) nl bulk
( ) nl gait
( ) nl ROM UE
( ) nl ROM LE
L___/5 UE R___/5
L___/5 LE R___/5

+ PE Findings

Assessment & Plan *remember your DDx!*

1.)

2.)

3.)

4.)

Labs

Notes

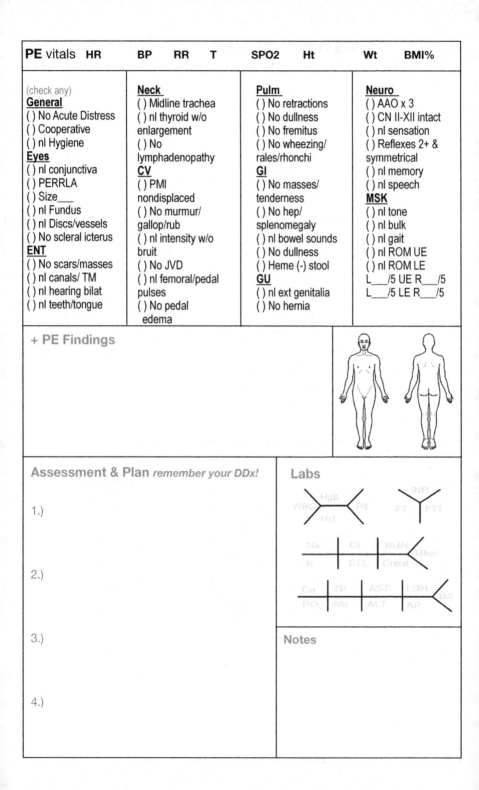

Date: **Initials/MRN:** **Age:** **Rotation:**

CC: _____ y/o M/F
HPI: *symptoms/pertinent +/- ROS/prior episodes/recent travel/sick contacts*

PMHx *child/adult illness /hospitalizations/ immunizations*

SurgHx *type/when/ why/complications*

FamHx *parents/siblings/ children*

SHx *smoker/ETOH/illicits/exercise/sex/maritalstatus*

Allergies *meds/foods/ environmental/reactions*

Meds *reason/dose/time/route/compliance/vitamins/ herbs/otcs*

ROS (circle any)

Gen
Fatigue
Weight +/-
Chills
Night sweats
Eyes
Pain
Redness
Vision changes
ENT
Headache
Hoarseness
Sore throat
Sinus sx
Hearing loss
Tinnitus
Runny nose

Pulm
Cough
SOB
Wheezing
Hemoptysis
CV
Chest pain
Edema
PND
Orthopnea
Palpitations
Claudication
GI
Abd pain
N/V
Heartburn
Bloody stools

GU
Dysuria
Frequency
Hematuria
Discharge
Flank pain
MS
Arthralgia
Arthritis
Joint swelling
Myalgias
Back pain
Heme
Bleeding
Bruising
Lymph
Swelling

Endo
Polyuria
Polydypsia
Polyphagia
Derm
Rash
Pruritis
Wound(s)
Neuro
Weakness
Seizures
Parasthesias
Tremors
Syncope
Psych
Anxiety
Depression

+ ROS Findings

PE vitals   **HR**   **BP**   **RR**   **T**   **SPO2**   **Ht**   **Wt**   **BMI%**

(check any)	**Neck**	**Pulm**	**Neuro**
General	( ) Midline trachea	( ) No retractions	( ) AAO x 3
( ) No Acute Distress	( ) nl thyroid w/o	( ) No dullness	( ) CN II-XII intact
( ) Cooperative	enlargement	( ) No fremitus	( ) nl sensation
( ) nl Hygiene	( ) No	( ) No wheezing/	( ) Reflexes 2+ &
Eyes	lymphadenopathy	rales/rhonchi	symmetrical
( ) nl conjunctiva	**CV**	**GI**	( ) nl memory
( ) PERRLA	( ) PMI	( ) No masses/	( ) nl speech
( ) Size___	nondisplaced	tenderness	**MSK**
( ) nl Fundus	( ) No murmur/	( ) No hep/	( ) nl tone
( ) nl Discs/vessels	gallop/rub	splenomegaly	( ) nl bulk
( ) No scleral icterus	( ) nl intensity w/o	( ) nl bowel sounds	( ) nl gait
ENT	bruit	( ) No dullness	( ) nl ROM UE
( ) No scars/masses	( ) No JVD	( ) Heme (-) stool	( ) nl ROM LE
( ) nl canals/ TM	( ) nl femoral/pedal	**GU**	L___/5 UE R___/5
( ) nl hearing bilat	pulses	( ) nl ext genitalia	L___/5 LE R___/5
( ) nl teeth/tongue	( ) No pedal	( ) No hernia	
	edema		

+ PE Findings

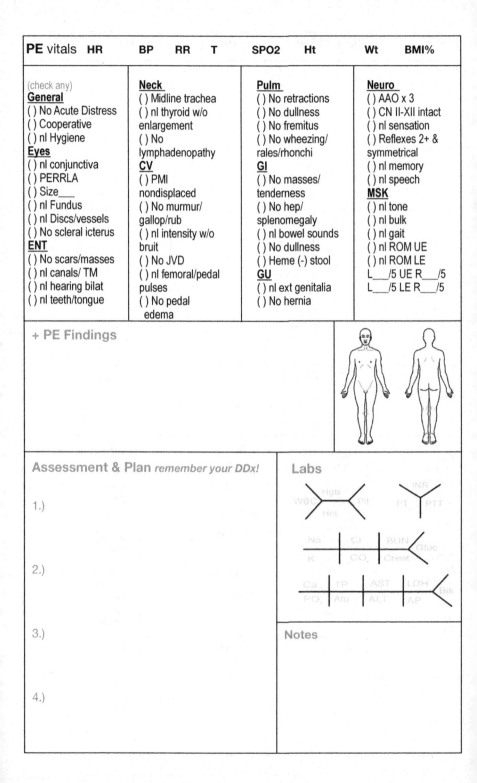

Assessment & Plan *remember your DDx!*

1.)

2.)

3.)

4.)

Labs

Notes

Date:	Initials/MRN:	Age:	Rotation:

CC: _____ y/o M/F
HPI: *symptoms/pertinent +/- ROS/prior episodes/recent travel/sick contacts*

PMHx *child/adult illness /hospitalizations/ immunizations*

SurgHx *type/when/ why/complications*

FamHx *parents/siblings/ children*

SHx *smoker/ETOH/illicits/exercise/sex/maritalstatus*

Allergies *meds/foods/ environmental/reactions*

Meds *reason/dose/time/route/compliance/vitamins/ herbs/otcs*

ROS (circle any)

Gen
Fatigue
Weight +/-
Chills
Night sweats
Eyes
Pain
Redness
Vision changes
ENT
Headache
Hoarseness
Sore throat
Sinus sx
Hearing loss
Tinnitus
Runny nose

Pulm
Cough
SOB
Wheezing
Hemoptysis
CV
Chest pain
Edema
PND
Orthopnea
Palpitations
Claudication
GI
Abd pain
N/V
Heartburn
Bloody stools

GU
Dysuria
Frequency
Hematuria
Discharge
Flank pain
MS
Arthralgia
Arthritis
Joint swelling
Myalgias
Back pain
Heme
Bleeding
Bruising
Lymph
Swelling

Endo
Polyuria
Polydypsia
Polyphagia
Derm
Rash
Pruritis
Wound(s)
Neuro
Weakness
Seizures
Parasthesias
Tremors
Syncope
Psych
Anxiety
Depression

+ ROS Findings

PE vitals **HR**   **BP**   **RR**   **T**   **SPO2**   **Ht**   **Wt**   **BMI%**

(check any)	**Neck**	**Pulm**	**Neuro**
General	( ) Midline trachea	( ) No retractions	( ) AAO x 3
( ) No Acute Distress	( ) nl thyroid w/o	( ) No dullness	( ) CN II-XII intact
( ) Cooperative	enlargement	( ) No fremitus	( ) nl sensation
( ) nl Hygiene	( ) No	( ) No wheezing/	( ) Reflexes 2+ &
Eyes	lymphadenopathy	rales/rhonchi	symmetrical
( ) nl conjunctiva	**CV**	**GI**	( ) nl memory
( ) PERRLA	( ) PMI	( ) No masses/	( ) nl speech
( ) Size___	nondisplaced	tenderness	**MSK**
( ) nl Fundus	( ) No murmur/	( ) No hep/	( ) nl tone
( ) nl Discs/vessels	gallop/rub	splenomegaly	( ) nl bulk
( ) No scleral icterus	( ) nl intensity w/o	( ) nl bowel sounds	( ) nl gait
ENT	bruit	( ) No dullness	( ) nl ROM UE
( ) No scars/masses	( ) No JVD	( ) Heme (-) stool	( ) nl ROM LE
( ) nl canals/ TM	( ) nl femoral/pedal	**GU**	L___/5 UE R___/5
( ) nl hearing bilat	pulses	( ) nl ext genitalia	L___/5 LE R___/5
( ) nl teeth/tongue	( ) No pedal	( ) No hernia	
	edema		

+ PE Findings

Assessment & Plan *remember your DDx!*

1.)

2.)

3.)

4.)

Labs

Notes

Date: **Initials/MRN:**   **Age:**   **Rotation:**

CC: _____ y/o M/F
HPI: *symptoms/pertinent +/- ROS/prior episodes/recent travel/sick contacts*

PMHx *child/adult illness /hospitalizations/ immunizations*

SurgHx *type/when/ why/complications*

FamHx *parents/siblings/ children*

SHx *smoker/ETOH/illicits/exercise/sex/maritalstatus*

Allergies *meds/foods/ environmental/reactions*

Meds *reason/dose/time/route/compliance/vitamins/ herbs/otcs*

ROS (circle any)

Gen
Fatigue
Weight +/-
Chills
Night sweats
Eyes
Pain
Redness
Vision changes
ENT
Headache
Hoarseness
Sore throat
Sinus sx
Hearing loss
Tinnitus
Runny nose

Pulm
Cough
SOB
Wheezing
Hemoptysis
CV
Chest pain
Edema
PND
Orthopnea
Palpitations
Claudication
GI
Abd pain
N/V
Heartburn
Bloody stools

GU
Dysuria
Frequency
Hematuria
Discharge
Flank pain
MS
Arthralgia
Arthritis
Joint swelling
Myalgias
Back pain
Heme
Bleeding
Bruising
Lymph
Swelling

Endo
Polyuria
Polydypsia
Polyphagia
Derm
Rash
Pruritis
Wound(s)
Neuro
Weakness
Seizures
Parasthesias
Tremors
Syncope
Psych
Anxiety
Depression

+ ROS Findings

PE vitals   **HR**   **BP**   **RR**   **T**   **SPO2**   **Ht**   **Wt**   **BMI%**

(check any)	**Neck**	**Pulm**	**Neuro**
General	( ) Midline trachea	( ) No retractions	( ) AAO x 3
( ) No Acute Distress	( ) nl thyroid w/o	( ) No dullness	( ) CN II-XII intact
( ) Cooperative	enlargement	( ) No fremitus	( ) nl sensation
( ) nl Hygiene	( ) No	( ) No wheezing/	( ) Reflexes 2+ &
Eyes	lymphadenopathy	rales/rhonchi	symmetrical
( ) nl conjunctiva	**CV**	**GI**	( ) nl memory
( ) PERRLA	( ) PMI	( ) No masses/	( ) nl speech
( ) Size___	nondisplaced	tenderness	**MSK**
( ) nl Fundus	( ) No murmur/	( ) No hep/	( ) nl tone
( ) nl Discs/vessels	gallop/rub	splenomegaly	( ) nl bulk
( ) No scleral icterus	( ) nl intensity w/o	( ) nl bowel sounds	( ) nl gait
ENT	bruit	( ) No dullness	( ) nl ROM UE
( ) No scars/masses	( ) No JVD	( ) Heme (-) stool	( ) nl ROM LE
( ) nl canals/ TM	( ) nl femoral/pedal	**GU**	L___/5 UE R___/5
( ) nl hearing bilat	pulses	( ) nl ext genitalia	L___/5 LE R___/5
( ) nl teeth/tongue	( ) No pedal	( ) No hernia	
	edema		

+ PE Findings

Assessment & Plan *remember your DDx!*

1.)

2.)

3.)

4.)

Labs

WBC Hgb Plt Hct

INR

PT PTT

Na Cl BUN
K CO₂ Creat Gluc

Ca TP AST LDH
PO₄ Alb ALT AP Bili

Notes

Date:	Initials/MRN:	Age:	Rotation:

CC: _____ y/o M/F
HPI: *symptoms/pertinent +/- ROS/prior episodes/recent travel/sick contacts*

PMHx *child/adult illness /hospitalizations/ immunizations*	**SurgHx** *type/when/ why/complications*	**FamHx** *parents/siblings/ children*

SHx *smoker/ETOH/illicits/exercise/sex/maritalstatus*

Allergies *meds/foods/ environmental/reactions*	**Meds** *reason/dose/time/route/compliance/vitamins/ herbs/otcs*

ROS (circle any)

Gen	**Pulm**	**GU**	**Endo**
Fatigue	Cough	Dysuria	Polyuria
Weight +/-	SOB	Frequency	Polydypsia
Chills	Wheezing	Hematuria	Polyphagia
Night sweats	Hemoptysis	Discharge	**Derm**
Eyes	**CV**	Flank pain	Rash
Pain	Chest pain	**MS**	Pruritis
Redness	Edema	Arthralgia	Wound(s)
Vision changes	PND	Arthritis	**Neuro**
ENT	Orthopnea	Joint swelling	Weakness
Headache	Palpitations	Myalgias	Seizures
Hoarseness	Claudication	Back pain	Parasthesias
Sore throat	**GI**	**Heme**	Tremors
Sinus sx	Abd pain	Bleeding	Syncope
Hearing loss	N/V	Bruising	**Psych**
Tinnitus	Heartburn	**Lymph**	Anxiety
Runny nose	Bloody stools	Swelling	Depression

+ ROS Findings

PE vitals   **HR**   **BP**   **RR**   **T**   **SPO2**   **Ht**   **Wt**   **BMI%**

(check any)

General
( ) No Acute Distress
( ) Cooperative
( ) nl Hygiene
Eyes
( ) nl conjunctiva
( ) PERRLA
( ) Size___
( ) nl Fundus
( ) nl Discs/vessels
( ) No scleral icterus
ENT
( ) No scars/masses
( ) nl canals/ TM
( ) nl hearing bilat
( ) nl teeth/tongue

Neck
( ) Midline trachea
( ) nl thyroid w/o
enlargement
( ) No
lymphadenopathy
CV
( ) PMI
nondisplaced
( ) No murmur/
gallop/rub
( ) nl intensity w/o
bruit
( ) No JVD
( ) nl femoral/pedal
pulses
( ) No pedal
edema

Pulm
( ) No retractions
( ) No dullness
( ) No fremitus
( ) No wheezing/
rales/rhonchi
GI
( ) No masses/
tenderness
( ) No hep/
splenomegaly
( ) nl bowel sounds
( ) No dullness
( ) Heme (-) stool
GU
( ) nl ext genitalia
( ) No hernia

Neuro
( ) AAO x 3
( ) CN II-XII intact
( ) nl sensation
( ) Reflexes 2+ &
symmetrical
( ) nl memory
( ) nl speech
MSK
( ) nl tone
( ) nl bulk
( ) nl gait
( ) nl ROM UE
( ) nl ROM LE
L___/5 UE R___/5
L___/5 LE R___/5

+ PE Findings

Assessment & Plan *remember your DDx!*

1.)

2.)

3.)

4.)

Labs

Notes

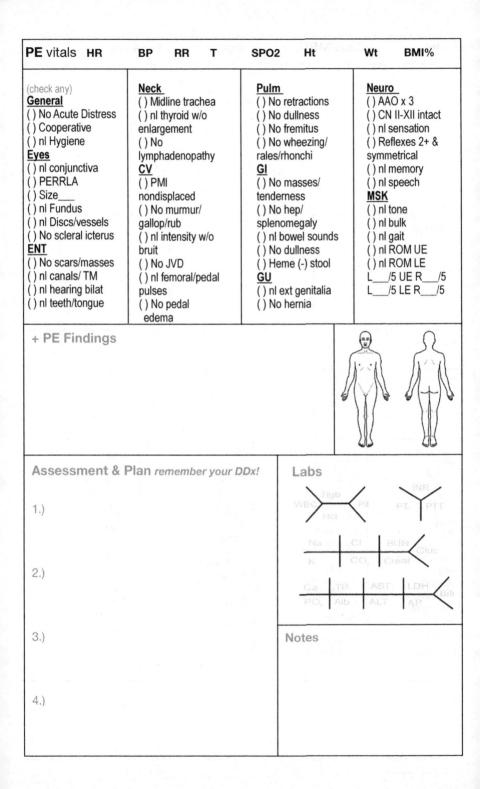

Date:	Initials/MRN:	Age:	Rotation:

CC: _____ y/o M/F
HPI: *symptoms/pertinent +/- ROS/prior episodes/recent travel/sick contacts*

PMHx *child/adult illness /hospitalizations/ immunizations*	**SurgHx** *type/when/ why/complications*	**FamHx** *parents/siblings/ children*

SHx *smoker/ETOH/illicits/exercise/sex/maritalstatus*

Allergies *meds/foods/ environmental/reactions*	**Meds** *reason/dose/time/route/compliance/vitamins/ herbs/otcs*

ROS (circle any)

Gen	**Pulm**	**GU**	**Endo**
Fatigue	Cough	Dysuria	Polyuria
Weight +/-	SOB	Frequency	Polydypsia
Chills	Wheezing	Hematuria	Polyphagia
Night sweats	Hemoptysis	Discharge	**Derm**
Eyes	**CV**	Flank pain	Rash
Pain	Chest pain	**MS**	Pruritis
Redness	Edema	Arthralgia	Wound(s)
Vision changes	PND	Arthritis	**Neuro**
ENT	Orthopnea	Joint swelling	Weakness
Headache	Palpitations	Myalgias	Seizures
Hoarseness	Claudication	Back pain	Parasthesias
Sore throat	**GI**	**Heme**	Tremors
Sinus sx	Abd pain	Bleeding	Syncope
Hearing loss	N/V	Bruising	**Psych**
Tinnitus	Heartburn	**Lymph**	Anxiety
Runny nose	Bloody stools	Swelling	Depression

+ ROS Findings

PE vitals	**HR**	**BP**	**RR**	**T**	**SPO2**	**Ht**	**Wt**	**BMI%**

(check any)

General
( ) No Acute Distress
( ) Cooperative
( ) nl Hygiene
Eyes
( ) nl conjunctiva
( ) PERRLA
( ) Size___
( ) nl Fundus
( ) nl Discs/vessels
( ) No scleral icterus
ENT
( ) No scars/masses
( ) nl canals/ TM
( ) nl hearing bilat
( ) nl teeth/tongue

Neck
( ) Midline trachea
( ) nl thyroid w/o
enlargement
( ) No
lymphadenopathy
CV
( ) PMI
nondisplaced
( ) No murmur/
gallop/rub
( ) nl intensity w/o
bruit
( ) No JVD
( ) nl femoral/pedal
pulses
( ) No pedal
edema

Pulm
( ) No retractions
( ) No dullness
( ) No fremitus
( ) No wheezing/
rales/rhonchi
GI
( ) No masses/
tenderness
( ) No hep/
splenomegaly
( ) nl bowel sounds
( ) No dullness
( ) Heme (-) stool
GU
( ) nl ext genitalia
( ) No hernia

Neuro
( ) AAO x 3
( ) CN II-XII intact
( ) nl sensation
( ) Reflexes 2+ &
symmetrical
( ) nl memory
( ) nl speech
MSK
( ) nl tone
( ) nl bulk
( ) nl gait
( ) nl ROM UE
( ) nl ROM LE
L___/5 UE R___/5
L___/5 LE R___/5

+ PE Findings

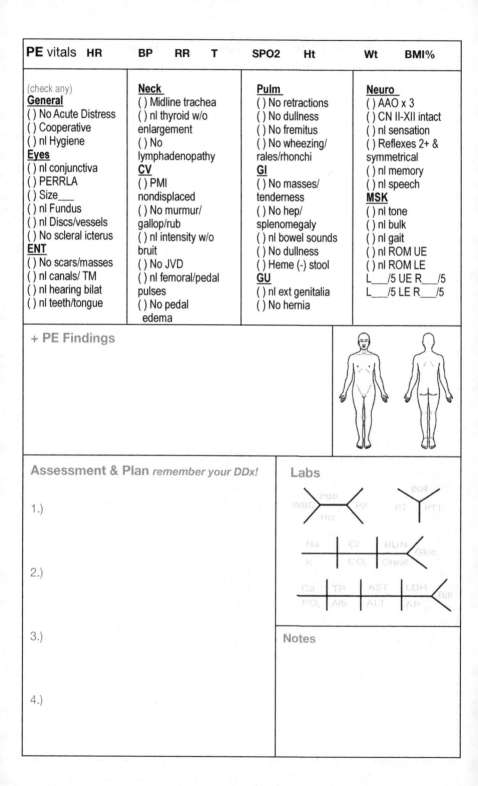

Assessment & Plan *remember your DDx!*

1.)

2.)

3.)

4.)

Labs

Notes

Date:	Initials/MRN:	Age:	Rotation:

CC: _____ y/o M/F
HPI: *symptoms/pertinent +/- ROS/prior episodes/recent travel/sick contacts*

PMHx *child/adult illness /hospitalizations/ immunizations*	**SurgHx** *type/when/ why/complications*	**FamHx** *parents/siblings/ children*

SHx *smoker/ETOH/illicits/exercise/sex/maritalstatus*

Allergies *meds/foods/ environmental/reactions*	**Meds** *reason/dose/time/route/compliance/vitamins/ herbs/otcs*

ROS (circle any)

Gen	**Pulm**	**GU**	**Endo**
Fatigue	Cough	Dysuria	Polyuria
Weight +/-	SOB	Frequency	Polydypsia
Chills	Wheezing	Hematuria	Polyphagia
Night sweats	Hemoptysis	Discharge	**Derm**
Eyes	**CV**	Flank pain	Rash
Pain	Chest pain	**MS**	Pruritis
Redness	Edema	Arthralgia	Wound(s)
Vision changes	PND	Arthritis	**Neuro**
ENT	Orthopnea	Joint swelling	Weakness
Headache	Palpitations	Myalgias	Seizures
Hoarseness	Claudication	Back pain	Parasthesias
Sore throat	**GI**	**Heme**	Tremors
Sinus sx	Abd pain	Bleeding	Syncope
Hearing loss	N/V	Bruising	**Psych**
Tinnitus	Heartburn	**Lymph**	Anxiety
Runny nose	Bloody stools	Swelling	Depression

+ ROS Findings

PE vitals	**HR**	**BP**	**RR**	**T**	**SPO2**	**Ht**	**Wt**	**BMI%**

(check any)	**Neck**	**Pulm**	**Neuro**
General	( ) Midline trachea	( ) No retractions	( ) AAO x 3
( ) No Acute Distress	( ) nl thyroid w/o	( ) No dullness	( ) CN II-XII intact
( ) Cooperative	enlargement	( ) No fremitus	( ) nl sensation
( ) nl Hygiene	( ) No	( ) No wheezing/	( ) Reflexes 2+ &
Eyes	lymphadenopathy	rales/rhonchi	symmetrical
( ) nl conjunctiva	**CV**	**GI**	( ) nl memory
( ) PERRLA	( ) PMI	( ) No masses/	( ) nl speech
( ) Size___	nondisplaced	tenderness	**MSK**
( ) nl Fundus	( ) No murmur/	( ) No hep/	( ) nl tone
( ) nl Discs/vessels	gallop/rub	splenomegaly	( ) nl bulk
( ) No scleral icterus	( ) nl intensity w/o	( ) nl bowel sounds	( ) nl gait
ENT	bruit	( ) No dullness	( ) nl ROM UE
( ) No scars/masses	( ) No JVD	( ) Heme (-) stool	( ) nl ROM LE
( ) nl canals/ TM	( ) nl femoral/pedal	**GU**	L___/5 UE R___/5
( ) nl hearing bilat	pulses	( ) nl ext genitalia	L___/5 LE R___/5
( ) nl teeth/tongue	( ) No pedal	( ) No hernia	
	edema		

+ PE Findings

Assessment & Plan *remember your DDx!*

1.)

2.)

3.)

4.)

Labs

Notes

Date:	Initials/MRN:	Age:	Rotation:

CC: _____ y/o M/F
HPI: *symptoms/pertinent +/- ROS/prior episodes/recent travel/sick contacts*

PMHx *child/adult illness /hospitalizations/ immunizations*	**SurgHx** *type/when/ why/complications*	**FamHx** *parents/siblings/ children*

SHx *smoker/ETOH/illicits/exercise/sex/maritalstatus*

Allergies *meds/foods/ environmental/reactions*	**Meds** *reason/dose/time/route/compliance/vitamins/ herbs/otcs*

ROS (circle any)

Gen	**Pulm**	**GU**	**Endo**
Fatigue	Cough	Dysuria	Polyuria
Weight +/-	SOB	Frequency	Polydypsia
Chills	Wheezing	Hematuria	Polyphagia
Night sweats	Hemoptysis	Discharge	**Derm**
Eyes	**CV**	Flank pain	Rash
Pain	Chest pain	**MS**	Pruritis
Redness	Edema	Arthralgia	Wound(s)
Vision changes	PND	Arthritis	**Neuro**
ENT	Orthopnea	Joint swelling	Weakness
Headache	Palpitations	Myalgias	Seizures
Hoarseness	Claudication	Back pain	Parasthesias
Sore throat	**GI**	**Heme**	Tremors
Sinus sx	Abd pain	Bleeding	Syncope
Hearing loss	N/V	Bruising	**Psych**
Tinnitus	Heartburn	**Lymph**	Anxiety
Runny nose	Bloody stools	Swelling	Depression

+ ROS Findings

PE vitals	HR	BP	RR	T	SPO2	Ht	Wt	BMI%

(check any)	**Neck**	**Pulm**	**Neuro**
General	( ) Midline trachea	( ) No retractions	( ) AAO x 3
( ) No Acute Distress	( ) nl thyroid w/o	( ) No dullness	( ) CN II-XII intact
( ) Cooperative	enlargement	( ) No fremitus	( ) nl sensation
( ) nl Hygiene	( ) No	( ) No wheezing/	( ) Reflexes 2+ &
Eyes	lymphadenopathy	rales/rhonchi	symmetrical
( ) nl conjunctiva	**CV**	**GI**	( ) nl memory
( ) PERRLA	( ) PMI	( ) No masses/	( ) nl speech
( ) Size___	nondisplaced	tenderness	**MSK**
( ) nl Fundus	( ) No murmur/	( ) No hep/	( ) nl tone
( ) nl Discs/vessels	gallop/rub	splenomegaly	( ) nl bulk
( ) No scleral icterus	( ) nl intensity w/o	( ) nl bowel sounds	( ) nl gait
ENT	bruit	( ) No dullness	( ) nl ROM UE
( ) No scars/masses	( ) No JVD	( ) Heme (-) stool	( ) nl ROM LE
( ) nl canals/ TM	( ) nl femoral/pedal	**GU**	L___/5 UE R___/5
( ) nl hearing bilat	pulses	( ) nl ext genitalia	L___/5 LE R___/5
( ) nl teeth/tongue	( ) No pedal	( ) No hernia	
	edema		

+ PE Findings

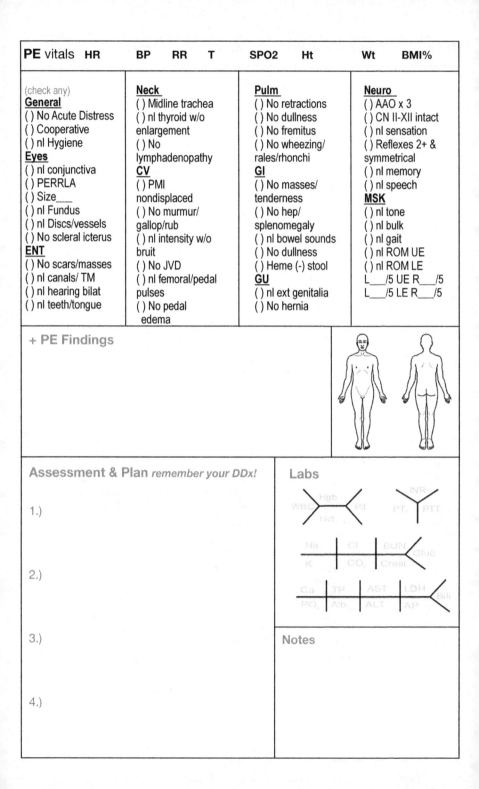

Assessment & Plan *remember your DDx!*

1.)

2.)

3.)

4.)

Labs

Notes

Date: **Initials/MRN:**   **Age:**   **Rotation:**

CC: _____ y/o M/F
HPI: *symptoms/pertinent +/- ROS/prior episodes/recent travel/sick contacts*

PMHx *child/adult illness /hospitalizations/ immunizations*	**SurgHx** *type/when/ why/complications*	**FamHx** *parents/siblings/ children*

SHx *smoker/ETOH/illicits/exercise/sex/maritalstatus*

Allergies *meds/foods/ environmental/reactions*	**Meds** *reason/dose/time/route/compliance/vitamins/ herbs/otcs*

ROS (circle any)

Gen	**Pulm**	**GU**	**Endo**
Fatigue	Cough	Dysuria	Polyuria
Weight +/-	SOB	Frequency	Polydypsia
Chills	Wheezing	Hematuria	Polyphagia
Night sweats	Hemoptysis	Discharge	**Derm**
Eyes	**CV**	Flank pain	Rash
Pain	Chest pain	**MS**	Pruritis
Redness	Edema	Arthralgia	Wound(s)
Vision changes	PND	Arthritis	**Neuro**
ENT	Orthopnea	Joint swelling	Weakness
Headache	Palpitations	Myalgias	Seizures
Hoarseness	Claudication	Back pain	Parasthesias
Sore throat	**GI**	**Heme**	Tremors
Sinus sx	Abd pain	Bleeding	Syncope
Hearing loss	N/V	Bruising	**Psych**
Tinnitus	Heartburn	**Lymph**	Anxiety
Runny nose	Bloody stools	Swelling	Depression

+ ROS Findings

PE vitals   HR   BP   RR   T   SPO2   Ht   Wt   BMI%

(check any) **General**	**Neck**	**Pulm**	**Neuro**
( ) No Acute Distress	( ) Midline trachea	( ) No retractions	( ) AAO x 3
( ) Cooperative	( ) nl thyroid w/o	( ) No dullness	( ) CN II-XII intact
( ) nl Hygiene	enlargement	( ) No fremitus	( ) nl sensation
Eyes	( ) No	( ) No wheezing/	( ) Reflexes 2+ &
( ) nl conjunctiva	lymphadenopathy	rales/rhonchi	symmetrical
( ) PERRLA	**CV**	**GI**	( ) nl memory
( ) Size___	( ) PMI	( ) No masses/	( ) nl speech
( ) nl Fundus	nondisplaced	tenderness	**MSK**
( ) nl Discs/vessels	( ) No murmur/	( ) No hep/	( ) nl tone
( ) No scleral icterus	gallop/rub	splenomegaly	( ) nl bulk
ENT	( ) nl intensity w/o	( ) nl bowel sounds	( ) nl gait
( ) No scars/masses	bruit	( ) No dullness	( ) nl ROM UE
( ) nl canals/ TM	( ) No JVD	( ) Heme (-) stool	( ) nl ROM LE
( ) nl hearing bilat	( ) nl femoral/pedal	**GU**	L___/5 UE R___/5
( ) nl teeth/tongue	pulses	( ) nl ext genitalia	L___/5 LE R___/5
	( ) No pedal	( ) No hernia	
	edema		

+ PE Findings

Assessment & Plan *remember your DDx!*

Labs

1.)

2.)

3.)

Notes

4.)

Date:	Initials/MRN:	Age:	Rotation:

CC: _____ y/o M/F
HPI: *symptoms/pertinent +/- ROS/prior episodes/recent travel/sick contacts*

PMHx *child/adult illness /hospitalizations/ immunizations*	**SurgHx** *type/when/ why/complications*	**FamHx** *parents/siblings/ children*

SHx *smoker/ETOH/illicits/exercise/sex/maritalstatus*

Allergies *meds/foods/ environmental/reactions*	**Meds** *reason/dose/time/route/compliance/vitamins/ herbs/otcs*

ROS (circle any)

Gen	**Pulm**	**GU**	**Endo**
Fatigue	Cough	Dysuria	Polyuria
Weight +/-	SOB	Frequency	Polydypsia
Chills	Wheezing	Hematuria	Polyphagia
Night sweats	Hemoptysis	Discharge	**Derm**
Eyes	**CV**	Flank pain	Rash
Pain	Chest pain	**MS**	Pruritis
Redness	Edema	Arthralgia	Wound(s)
Vision changes	PND	Arthritis	**Neuro**
ENT	Orthopnea	Joint swelling	Weakness
Headache	Palpitations	Myalgias	Seizures
Hoarseness	Claudication	Back pain	Parasthesias
Sore throat	**GI**	**Heme**	Tremors
Sinus sx	Abd pain	Bleeding	Syncope
Hearing loss	N/V	Bruising	**Psych**
Tinnitus	Heartburn	**Lymph**	Anxiety
Runny nose	Bloody stools	Swelling	Depression

+ ROS Findings

PE vitals   **HR**   **BP**   **RR**   **T**   **SPO2**   **Ht**   **Wt**   **BMI%**

(check any)

General
( ) No Acute Distress
( ) Cooperative
( ) nl Hygiene
Eyes
( ) nl conjunctiva
( ) PERRLA
( ) Size___
( ) nl Fundus
( ) nl Discs/vessels
( ) No scleral icterus
ENT
( ) No scars/masses
( ) nl canals/ TM
( ) nl hearing bilat
( ) nl teeth/tongue

Neck
( ) Midline trachea
( ) nl thyroid w/o
enlargement
( ) No
lymphadenopathy
CV
( ) PMI
nondisplaced
( ) No murmur/
gallop/rub
( ) nl intensity w/o
bruit
( ) No JVD
( ) nl femoral/pedal
pulses
( ) No pedal
edema

Pulm
( ) No retractions
( ) No dullness
( ) No fremitus
( ) No wheezing/
rales/rhonchi
GI
( ) No masses/
tenderness
( ) No hep/
splenomegaly
( ) nl bowel sounds
( ) No dullness
( ) Heme (-) stool
GU
( ) nl ext genitalia
( ) No hernia

Neuro
( ) AAO x 3
( ) CN II-XII intact
( ) nl sensation
( ) Reflexes 2+ &
symmetrical
( ) nl memory
( ) nl speech
MSK
( ) nl tone
( ) nl bulk
( ) nl gait
( ) nl ROM UE
( ) nl ROM LE
L___/5 UE R___/5
L___/5 LE R___/5

+ PE Findings

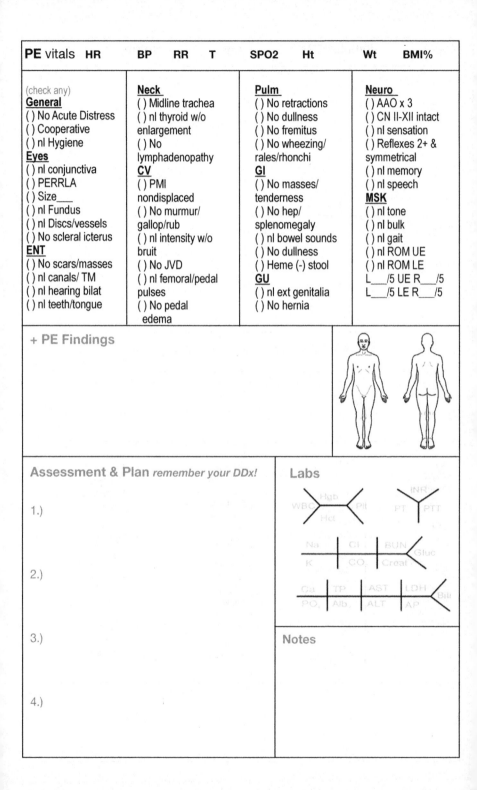

Assessment & Plan *remember your DDx!*

1.)

2.)

3.)

4.)

Labs

WBC   Hgb   Plt   INR   PT   PTT
    Hct

Na   Cl   BUN   Gluc
K   CO₂   Creat

Ca   TP   AST   LDH   Bili
PO₄   Alb   ALT   AP

Notes

Date:	Initials/MRN:	Age:	Rotation:

CC: _____ y/o M/F
HPI: *symptoms/pertinent +/- ROS/prior episodes/recent travel/sick contacts*

PMHx *child/adult illness /hospitalizations/ immunizations*

SurgHx *type/when/ why/complications*

FamHx *parents/siblings/ children*

SHx *smoker/ETOH/illicits/exercise/sex/maritalstatus*

Allergies *meds/foods/ environmental/reactions*

Meds *reason/dose/time/route/compliance/vitamins/ herbs/otcs*

ROS (circle any)

Gen
Fatigue
Weight +/-
Chills
Night sweats
Eyes
Pain
Redness
Vision changes
ENT
Headache
Hoarseness
Sore throat
Sinus sx
Hearing loss
Tinnitus
Runny nose

Pulm
Cough
SOB
Wheezing
Hemoptysis
CV
Chest pain
Edema
PND
Orthopnea
Palpitations
Claudication
GI
Abd pain
N/V
Heartburn
Bloody stools

GU
Dysuria
Frequency
Hematuria
Discharge
Flank pain
MS
Arthralgia
Arthritis
Joint swelling
Myalgias
Back pain
Heme
Bleeding
Bruising
Lymph
Swelling

Endo
Polyuria
Polydypsia
Polyphagia
Derm
Rash
Pruritis
Wound(s)
Neuro
Weakness
Seizures
Parasthesias
Tremors
Syncope
Psych
Anxiety
Depression

+ ROS Findings

PE vitals   **HR**   **BP**   **RR**   **T**   **SPO2**   **Ht**   **Wt**   **BMI%**

(check any)	**Neck**	**Pulm**	**Neuro**
General	( ) Midline trachea	( ) No retractions	( ) AAO x 3
( ) No Acute Distress	( ) nl thyroid w/o	( ) No dullness	( ) CN II-XII intact
( ) Cooperative	enlargement	( ) No fremitus	( ) nl sensation
( ) nl Hygiene	( ) No	( ) No wheezing/	( ) Reflexes 2+ &
Eyes	lymphadenopathy	rales/rhonchi	symmetrical
( ) nl conjunctiva	**CV**	**GI**	( ) nl memory
( ) PERRLA	( ) PMI	( ) No masses/	( ) nl speech
( ) Size___	nondisplaced	tenderness	**MSK**
( ) nl Fundus	( ) No murmur/	( ) No hep/	( ) nl tone
( ) nl Discs/vessels	gallop/rub	splenomegaly	( ) nl bulk
( ) No scleral icterus	( ) nl intensity w/o	( ) nl bowel sounds	( ) nl gait
ENT	bruit	( ) No dullness	( ) nl ROM UE
( ) No scars/masses	( ) No JVD	( ) Heme (-) stool	( ) nl ROM LE
( ) nl canals/ TM	( ) nl femoral/pedal	**GU**	L___/5 UE R___/5
( ) nl hearing bilat	pulses	( ) nl ext genitalia	L___/5 LE R___/5
( ) nl teeth/tongue	( ) No pedal	( ) No hernia	
	edema		

+ PE Findings

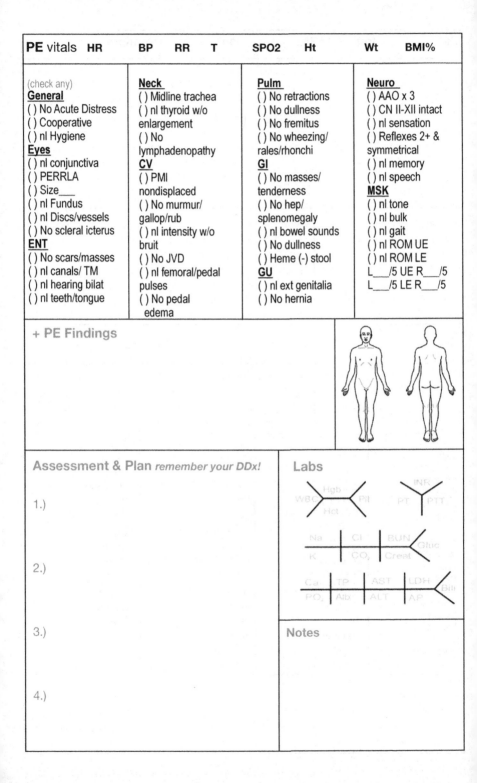

Assessment & Plan *remember your DDx!*

1.)

2.)

3.)

4.)

Labs

Notes

Date:	Initials/MRN:	Age:	Rotation:

CC: _____ y/o M/F
HPI: *symptoms/pertinent +/- ROS/prior episodes/recent travel/sick contacts*

PMHx *child/adult illness /hospitalizations/ immunizations*

SurgHx *type/when/ why/complications*

FamHx *parents/siblings/ children*

SHx *smoker/ETOH/illicits/exercise/sex/maritalstatus*

Allergies *meds/foods/ environmental/reactions*

Meds *reason/dose/time/route/compliance/vitamins/ herbs/otcs*

ROS (circle any)

Gen
Fatigue
Weight +/-
Chills
Night sweats
Eyes
Pain
Redness
Vision changes
ENT
Headache
Hoarseness
Sore throat
Sinus sx
Hearing loss
Tinnitus
Runny nose

Pulm
Cough
SOB
Wheezing
Hemoptysis
CV
Chest pain
Edema
PND
Orthopnea
Palpitations
Claudication
GI
Abd pain
N/V
Heartburn
Bloody stools

GU
Dysuria
Frequency
Hematuria
Discharge
Flank pain
MS
Arthralgia
Arthritis
Joint swelling
Myalgias
Back pain
Heme
Bleeding
Bruising
Lymph
Swelling

Endo
Polyuria
Polydypsia
Polyphagia
Derm
Rash
Pruritis
Wound(s)
Neuro
Weakness
Seizures
Parasthesias
Tremors
Syncope
Psych
Anxiety
Depression

+ ROS Findings

PE vitals	**HR**	**BP**	**RR**	**T**	**SPO2**	**Ht**	**Wt**	**BMI%**

(check any)

General
( ) No Acute Distress
( ) Cooperative
( ) nl Hygiene
Eyes
( ) nl conjunctiva
( ) PERRLA
( ) Size___
( ) nl Fundus
( ) nl Discs/vessels
( ) No scleral icterus
ENT
( ) No scars/masses
( ) nl canals/ TM
( ) nl hearing bilat
( ) nl teeth/tongue

Neck
( ) Midline trachea
( ) nl thyroid w/o
enlargement
( ) No
lymphadenopathy
CV
( ) PMI
nondisplaced
( ) No murmur/
gallop/rub
( ) nl intensity w/o
bruit
( ) No JVD
( ) nl femoral/pedal
pulses
( ) No pedal
edema

Pulm
( ) No retractions
( ) No dullness
( ) No fremitus
( ) No wheezing/
rales/rhonchi
GI
( ) No masses/
tenderness
( ) No hep/
splenomegaly
( ) nl bowel sounds
( ) No dullness
( ) Heme (-) stool
GU
( ) nl ext genitalia
( ) No hernia

Neuro
( ) AAO x 3
( ) CN II-XII intact
( ) nl sensation
( ) Reflexes 2+ &
symmetrical
( ) nl memory
( ) nl speech
MSK
( ) nl tone
( ) nl bulk
( ) nl gait
( ) nl ROM UE
( ) nl ROM LE
L___/5 UE R___/5
L___/5 LE R___/5

+ PE Findings

Assessment & Plan *remember your DDx!*

1.)

2.)

3.)

4.)

Labs

Notes

Date:	Initials/MRN:	Age:	Rotation:

CC: _____ y/o M/F
HPI: *symptoms/pertinent +/- ROS/prior episodes/recent travel/sick contacts*

PMHx *child/adult illness /hospitalizations/ immunizations*	**SurgHx** *type/when/ why/complications*	**FamHx** *parents/siblings/ children*

SHx *smoker/ETOH/illicits/exercise/sex/maritalstatus*

Allergies *meds/foods/ environmental/reactions*	**Meds** *reason/dose/time/route/compliance/vitamins/ herbs/otcs*

ROS (circle any)

Gen	**Pulm**	**GU**	**Endo**
Fatigue	Cough	Dysuria	Polyuria
Weight +/-	SOB	Frequency	Polydypsia
Chills	Wheezing	Hematuria	Polyphagia
Night sweats	Hemoptysis	Discharge	**Derm**
Eyes	**CV**	Flank pain	Rash
Pain	Chest pain	**MS**	Pruritis
Redness	Edema	Arthralgia	Wound(s)
Vision changes	PND	Arthritis	**Neuro**
ENT	Orthopnea	Joint swelling	Weakness
Headache	Palpitations	Myalgias	Seizures
Hoarseness	Claudication	Back pain	Parasthesias
Sore throat	**GI**	**Heme**	Tremors
Sinus sx	Abd pain	Bleeding	Syncope
Hearing loss	N/V	Bruising	**Psych**
Tinnitus	Heartburn	**Lymph**	Anxiety
Runny nose	Bloody stools	Swelling	Depression

+ ROS Findings

PE vitals HR   BP   RR   T   SPO2   Ht   Wt   BMI%

(check any) **General** ( ) No Acute Distress ( ) Cooperative ( ) nl Hygiene **Eyes** ( ) nl conjunctiva ( ) PERRLA ( ) Size___ ( ) nl Fundus ( ) nl Discs/vessels ( ) No scleral icterus **ENT** ( ) No scars/masses ( ) nl canals/ TM ( ) nl hearing bilat ( ) nl teeth/tongue	**Neck** ( ) Midline trachea ( ) nl thyroid w/o enlargement ( ) No lymphadenopathy **CV** ( ) PMI nondisplaced ( ) No murmur/ gallop/rub ( ) nl intensity w/o bruit ( ) No JVD ( ) nl femoral/pedal pulses ( ) No pedal edema	**Pulm** ( ) No retractions ( ) No dullness ( ) No fremitus ( ) No wheezing/ rales/rhonchi **GI** ( ) No masses/ tenderness ( ) No hep/ splenomegaly ( ) nl bowel sounds ( ) No dullness ( ) Heme (-) stool **GU** ( ) nl ext genitalia ( ) No hernia	**Neuro** ( ) AAO x 3 ( ) CN II-XII intact ( ) nl sensation ( ) Reflexes 2+ & symmetrical ( ) nl memory ( ) nl speech **MSK** ( ) nl tone ( ) nl bulk ( ) nl gait ( ) nl ROM UE ( ) nl ROM LE L___/5 UE R___/5 L___/5 LE R___/5

+ PE Findings

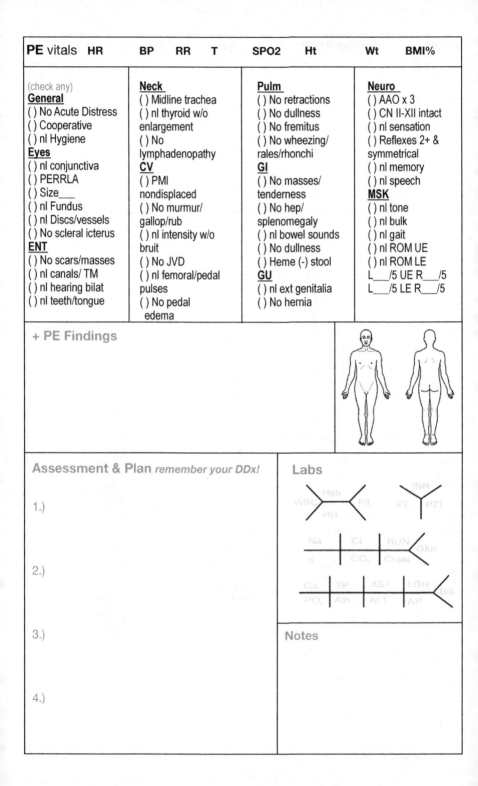

Assessment & Plan *remember your DDx!*

1.)

2.)

3.)

4.)

Labs

Notes

Date:	Initials/MRN:	Age:	Rotation:

CC: _____ y/o M/F
HPI: *symptoms/pertinent +/- ROS/prior episodes/recent travel/sick contacts*

PMHx *child/adult illness /hospitalizations/ immunizations*	**SurgHx** *type/when/ why/complications*	**FamHx** *parents/siblings/ children*

SHx *smoker/ETOH/illicits/exercise/sex/maritalstatus*

Allergies *meds/foods/ environmental/reactions*	**Meds** *reason/dose/time/route/compliance/vitamins/ herbs/otcs*

ROS (circle any)

Gen	**Pulm**	**GU**	**Endo**
Fatigue	Cough	Dysuria	Polyuria
Weight +/-	SOB	Frequency	Polydypsia
Chills	Wheezing	Hematuria	Polyphagia
Night sweats	Hemoptysis	Discharge	**Derm**
Eyes	**CV**	Flank pain	Rash
Pain	Chest pain	**MS**	Pruritis
Redness	Edema	Arthralgia	Wound(s)
Vision changes	PND	Arthritis	**Neuro**
ENT	Orthopnea	Joint swelling	Weakness
Headache	Palpitations	Myalgias	Seizures
Hoarseness	Claudication	Back pain	Parasthesias
Sore throat	**GI**	**Heme**	Tremors
Sinus sx	Abd pain	Bleeding	Syncope
Hearing loss	N/V	Bruising	**Psych**
Tinnitus	Heartburn	**Lymph**	Anxiety
Runny nose	Bloody stools	Swelling	Depression

+ ROS Findings

PE vitals **HR**   **BP**   **RR**   **T**   **SPO2**   **Ht**   **Wt**   **BMI%**

(check any)	**Neck**	**Pulm**	**Neuro**
General	( ) Midline trachea	( ) No retractions	( ) AAO x 3
( ) No Acute Distress	( ) nl thyroid w/o	( ) No dullness	( ) CN II-XII intact
( ) Cooperative	enlargement	( ) No fremitus	( ) nl sensation
( ) nl Hygiene	( ) No	( ) No wheezing/	( ) Reflexes 2+ &
Eyes	lymphadenopathy	rales/rhonchi	symmetrical
( ) nl conjunctiva	**CV**	**GI**	( ) nl memory
( ) PERRLA	( ) PMI	( ) No masses/	( ) nl speech
( ) Size___	nondisplaced	tenderness	**MSK**
( ) nl Fundus	( ) No murmur/	( ) No hep/	( ) nl tone
( ) nl Discs/vessels	gallop/rub	splenomegaly	( ) nl bulk
( ) No scleral icterus	( ) nl intensity w/o	( ) nl bowel sounds	( ) nl gait
ENT	bruit	( ) No dullness	( ) nl ROM UE
( ) No scars/masses	( ) No JVD	( ) Heme (-) stool	( ) nl ROM LE
( ) nl canals/ TM	( ) nl femoral/pedal	**GU**	L___/5 UE R___/5
( ) nl hearing bilat	pulses	( ) nl ext genitalia	L___/5 LE R___/5
( ) nl teeth/tongue	( ) No pedal	( ) No hernia	
	edema		

+ PE Findings

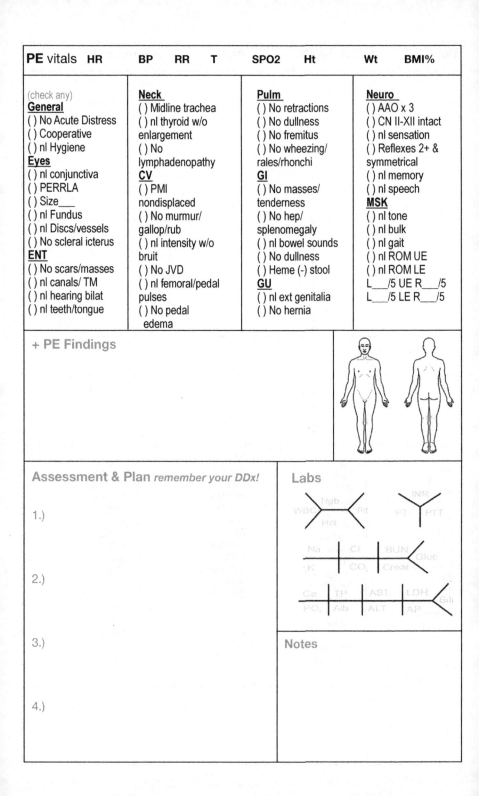

Assessment & Plan *remember your DDx!*

1.)

2.)

3.)

4.)

Labs

Notes

Date:	Initials/MRN:	Age:	Rotation:

CC: _____ y/o M/F
HPI: *symptoms/pertinent +/- ROS/prior episodes/recent travel/sick contacts*

PMHx *child/adult illness /hospitalizations/ immunizations*	**SurgHx** *type/when/ why/complications*	**FamHx** *parents/siblings/ children*

SHx *smoker/ETOH/illicits/exercise/sex/maritalstatus*

Allergies *meds/foods/ environmental/reactions*	**Meds** *reason/dose/time/route/compliance/vitamins/ herbs/otcs*

ROS (circle any)

Gen Fatigue Weight +/- Chills Night sweats **Eyes** Pain Redness Vision changes **ENT** Headache Hoarseness Sore throat Sinus sx Hearing loss Tinnitus Runny nose	**Pulm** Cough SOB Wheezing Hemoptysis **CV** Chest pain Edema PND Orthopnea Palpitations Claudication **GI** Abd pain N/V Heartburn Bloody stools	**GU** Dysuria Frequency Hematuria Discharge Flank pain **MS** Arthralgia Arthritis Joint swelling Myalgias Back pain **Heme** Bleeding Bruising **Lymph** Swelling	**Endo** Polyuria Polydypsia Polyphagia **Derm** Rash Pruritis Wound(s) **Neuro** Weakness Seizures Parasthesias Tremors Syncope **Psych** Anxiety Depression

+ ROS Findings

PE vitals	HR	BP	RR	T	SPO2	Ht	Wt	BMI%

(check any) **General**	**Neck**	**Pulm**	**Neuro**
( ) No Acute Distress	( ) Midline trachea	( ) No retractions	( ) AAO x 3
( ) Cooperative	( ) nl thyroid w/o	( ) No dullness	( ) CN II-XII intact
( ) nl Hygiene	enlargement	( ) No fremitus	( ) nl sensation
Eyes	( ) No	( ) No wheezing/	( ) Reflexes 2+ &
( ) nl conjunctiva	lymphadenopathy	rales/rhonchi	symmetrical
( ) PERRLA	**CV**	**GI**	( ) nl memory
( ) Size___	( ) PMI	( ) No masses/	( ) nl speech
( ) nl Fundus	nondisplaced	tenderness	**MSK**
( ) nl Discs/vessels	( ) No murmur/	( ) No hep/	( ) nl tone
( ) No scleral icterus	gallop/rub	splenomegaly	( ) nl bulk
ENT	( ) nl intensity w/o	( ) nl bowel sounds	( ) nl gait
( ) No scars/masses	bruit	( ) No dullness	( ) nl ROM UE
( ) nl canals/ TM	( ) No JVD	( ) Heme (-) stool	( ) nl ROM LE
( ) nl hearing bilat	( ) nl femoral/pedal	**GU**	L___/5 UE R___/5
( ) nl teeth/tongue	pulses	( ) nl ext genitalia	L___/5 LE R___/5
	( ) No pedal	( ) No hernia	
	edema		

+ PE Findings

Assessment & Plan *remember your DDx!*

1.)

2.)

3.)

4.)

Labs

Notes

Date:	Initials/MRN:	Age:	Rotation:

CC: _____ y/o M/F
HPI: *symptoms/pertinent +/- ROS/prior episodes/recent travel/sick contacts*

PMHx *child/adult illness /hospitalizations/ immunizations*	**SurgHx** *type/when/ why/complications*	**FamHx** *parents/siblings/ children*

SHx *smoker/ETOH/illicits/exercise/sex/maritalstatus*

Allergies *meds/foods/ environmental/reactions*	**Meds** *reason/dose/time/route/compliance/vitamins/ herbs/otcs*

ROS (circle any)

Gen	**Pulm**	**GU**	**Endo**
Fatigue	Cough	Dysuria	Polyuria
Weight +/-	SOB	Frequency	Polydypsia
Chills	Wheezing	Hematuria	Polyphagia
Night sweats	Hemoptysis	Discharge	**Derm**
Eyes	**CV**	Flank pain	Rash
Pain	Chest pain	**MS**	Pruritis
Redness	Edema	Arthralgia	Wound(s)
Vision changes	PND	Arthritis	**Neuro**
ENT	Orthopnea	Joint swelling	Weakness
Headache	Palpitations	Myalgias	Seizures
Hoarseness	Claudication	Back pain	Parasthesias
Sore throat	**GI**	**Heme**	Tremors
Sinus sx	Abd pain	Bleeding	Syncope
Hearing loss	N/V	Bruising	**Psych**
Tinnitus	Heartburn	**Lymph**	Anxiety
Runny nose	Bloody stools	Swelling	Depression

+ ROS Findings

PE vitals   HR   BP   RR   T   SPO2   Ht   Wt   BMI%

(check any) **General**	**Neck**	**Pulm**	**Neuro**
( ) No Acute Distress	( ) Midline trachea	( ) No retractions	( ) AAO x 3
( ) Cooperative	( ) nl thyroid w/o	( ) No dullness	( ) CN II-XII intact
( ) nl Hygiene	enlargement	( ) No fremitus	( ) nl sensation
Eyes	( ) No	( ) No wheezing/	( ) Reflexes 2+ &
( ) nl conjunctiva	lymphadenopathy	rales/rhonchi	symmetrical
( ) PERRLA	**CV**	**GI**	( ) nl memory
( ) Size___	( ) PMI	( ) No masses/	( ) nl speech
( ) nl Fundus	nondisplaced	tenderness	**MSK**
( ) nl Discs/vessels	( ) No murmur/	( ) No hep/	( ) nl tone
( ) No scleral icterus	gallop/rub	splenomegaly	( ) nl bulk
ENT	( ) nl intensity w/o	( ) nl bowel sounds	( ) nl gait
( ) No scars/masses	bruit	( ) No dullness	( ) nl ROM UE
( ) nl canals/ TM	( ) No JVD	( ) Heme (-) stool	( ) nl ROM LE
( ) nl hearing bilat	( ) nl femoral/pedal	**GU**	L___/5 UE R___/5
( ) nl teeth/tongue	pulses	( ) nl ext genitalia	L___/5 LE R___/5
	( ) No pedal	( ) No hernia	
	edema		

+ PE Findings

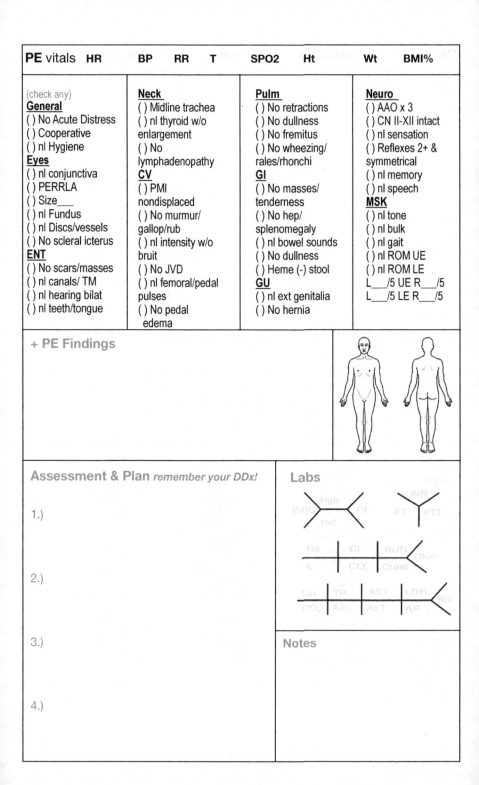

Assessment & Plan *remember your DDx!*

1.)

2.)

3.)

4.)

Labs

WBC   Hgb   Plt   INR   PT   PTT
Hct

Na   Cl   BUN   Gluc
K   CO₂   Creat

Ca   TP   AST   LDH   Bili
PO₄   Alb   ALT   AP

Notes

Date:	Initials/MRN:	Age:	Rotation:

CC: _____ y/o M/F
HPI: *symptoms/pertinent +/- ROS/prior episodes/recent travel/sick contacts*

PMHx *child/adult illness /hospitalizations/ immunizations*	**SurgHx** *type/when/ why/complications*	**FamHx** *parents/siblings/ children*

SHx *smoker/ETOH/illicits/exercise/sex/maritalstatus*

Allergies *meds/foods/ environmental/reactions*	**Meds** *reason/dose/time/route/compliance/vitamins/ herbs/otcs*

ROS (circle any)

Gen	**Pulm**	**GU**	**Endo**
Fatigue	Cough	Dysuria	Polyuria
Weight +/-	SOB	Frequency	Polydypsia
Chills	Wheezing	Hematuria	Polyphagia
Night sweats	Hemoptysis	Discharge	**Derm**
Eyes	**CV**	Flank pain	Rash
Pain	Chest pain	**MS**	Pruritis
Redness	Edema	Arthralgia	Wound(s)
Vision changes	PND	Arthritis	**Neuro**
ENT	Orthopnea	Joint swelling	Weakness
Headache	Palpitations	Myalgias	Seizures
Hoarseness	Claudication	Back pain	Parasthesias
Sore throat	**GI**	**Heme**	Tremors
Sinus sx	Abd pain	Bleeding	Syncope
Hearing loss	N/V	Bruising	**Psych**
Tinnitus	Heartburn	**Lymph**	Anxiety
Runny nose	Bloody stools	Swelling	Depression

+ ROS Findings

PE vitals HR	BP RR T	SPO2 Ht	Wt BMI%

(check any)	**Neck**	**Pulm**	**Neuro**
General	( ) Midline trachea	( ) No retractions	( ) AAO x 3
( ) No Acute Distress	( ) nl thyroid w/o	( ) No dullness	( ) CN II-XII intact
( ) Cooperative	enlargement	( ) No fremitus	( ) nl sensation
( ) nl Hygiene	( ) No	( ) No wheezing/	( ) Reflexes 2+ &
Eyes	lymphadenopathy	rales/rhonchi	symmetrical
( ) nl conjunctiva	**CV**	**GI**	( ) nl memory
( ) PERRLA	( ) PMI	( ) No masses/	( ) nl speech
( ) Size___	nondisplaced	tenderness	**MSK**
( ) nl Fundus	( ) No murmur/	( ) No hep/	( ) nl tone
( ) nl Discs/vessels	gallop/rub	splenomegaly	( ) nl bulk
( ) No scleral icterus	( ) nl intensity w/o	( ) nl bowel sounds	( ) nl gait
ENT	bruit	( ) No dullness	( ) nl ROM UE
( ) No scars/masses	( ) No JVD	( ) Heme (-) stool	( ) nl ROM LE
( ) nl canals/ TM	( ) nl femoral/pedal	**GU**	L___/5 UE R___/5
( ) nl hearing bilat	pulses	( ) nl ext genitalia	L___/5 LE R___/5
( ) nl teeth/tongue	( ) No pedal	( ) No hernia	
	edema		

+ PE Findings

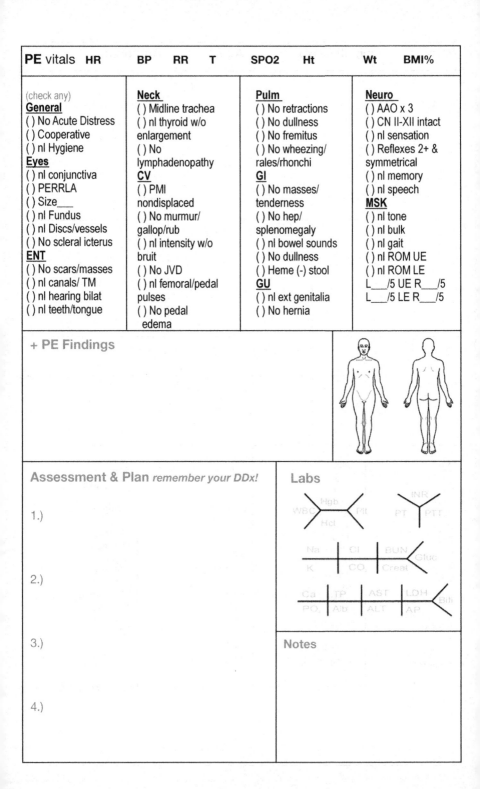

Assessment & Plan *remember your DDx!*

1.)

2.)

3.)

4.)

Labs

Notes

Date:	Initials/MRN:	Age:	Rotation:

CC: _____ y/o M/F
HPI: *symptoms/pertinent +/- ROS/prior episodes/recent travel/sick contacts*

PMHx *child/adult illness /hospitalizations/ immunizations*

SurgHx *type/when/ why/complications*

FamHx *parents/siblings/ children*

SHx *smoker/ETOH/illicits/exercise/sex/maritalstatus*

Allergies *meds/foods/ environmental/reactions*

Meds *reason/dose/time/route/compliance/vitamins/ herbs/otcs*

ROS (circle any)

Gen	**Pulm**	**GU**	**Endo**
Fatigue	Cough	Dysuria	Polyuria
Weight +/-	SOB	Frequency	Polydypsia
Chills	Wheezing	Hematuria	Polyphagia
Night sweats	Hemoptysis	Discharge	**Derm**
Eyes	**CV**	Flank pain	Rash
Pain	Chest pain	**MS**	Pruritis
Redness	Edema	Arthralgia	Wound(s)
Vision changes	PND	Arthritis	**Neuro**
ENT	Orthopnea	Joint swelling	Weakness
Headache	Palpitations	Myalgias	Seizures
Hoarseness	Claudication	Back pain	Parasthesias
Sore throat	**GI**	**Heme**	Tremors
Sinus sx	Abd pain	Bleeding	Syncope
Hearing loss	N/V	Bruising	**Psych**
Tinnitus	Heartburn	**Lymph**	Anxiety
Runny nose	Bloody stools	Swelling	Depression

+ ROS Findings

PE vitals   **HR**   **BP**   **RR**   **T**   **SPO2**   **Ht**   **Wt**   **BMI%**

(check any) **General** ( ) No Acute Distress ( ) Cooperative ( ) nl Hygiene **Eyes** ( ) nl conjunctiva ( ) PERRLA ( ) Size___ ( ) nl Fundus ( ) nl Discs/vessels ( ) No scleral icterus **ENT** ( ) No scars/masses ( ) nl canals/ TM ( ) nl hearing bilat ( ) nl teeth/tongue	**Neck** ( ) Midline trachea ( ) nl thyroid w/o enlargement ( ) No lymphadenopathy **CV** ( ) PMI nondisplaced ( ) No murmur/ gallop/rub ( ) nl intensity w/o bruit ( ) No JVD ( ) nl femoral/pedal pulses ( ) No pedal edema	**Pulm** ( ) No retractions ( ) No dullness ( ) No fremitus ( ) No wheezing/ rales/rhonchi **GI** ( ) No masses/ tenderness ( ) No hep/ splenomegaly ( ) nl bowel sounds ( ) No dullness ( ) Heme (-) stool **GU** ( ) nl ext genitalia ( ) No hernia	**Neuro** ( ) AAO x 3 ( ) CN II-XII intact ( ) nl sensation ( ) Reflexes 2+ & symmetrical ( ) nl memory ( ) nl speech **MSK** ( ) nl tone ( ) nl bulk ( ) nl gait ( ) nl ROM UE ( ) nl ROM LE L___/5 UE R___/5 L___/5 LE R___/5

+ PE Findings

Assessment & Plan *remember your DDx!*

1.)

2.)

3.)

4.)

Labs

Notes

Date:	Initials/MRN:	Age:	Rotation:

CC: _____ y/o M/F
HPI: *symptoms/pertinent +/- ROS/prior episodes/recent travel/sick contacts*

PMHx *child/adult illness /hospitalizations/ immunizations*	**SurgHx** *type/when/ why/complications*	**FamHx** *parents/siblings/ children*

SHx *smoker/ETOH/illicits/exercise/sex/maritalstatus*

Allergies *meds/foods/ environmental/reactions*	**Meds** *reason/dose/time/route/compliance/vitamins/ herbs/otcs*

ROS (circle any)

Gen	**Pulm**	**GU**	**Endo**
Fatigue	Cough	Dysuria	Polyuria
Weight +/-	SOB	Frequency	Polydypsia
Chills	Wheezing	Hematuria	Polyphagia
Night sweats	Hemoptysis	Discharge	**Derm**
Eyes	**CV**	Flank pain	Rash
Pain	Chest pain	**MS**	Pruritis
Redness	Edema	Arthralgia	Wound(s)
Vision changes	PND	Arthritis	**Neuro**
ENT	Orthopnea	Joint swelling	Weakness
Headache	Palpitations	Myalgias	Seizures
Hoarseness	Claudication	Back pain	Parasthesias
Sore throat	**GI**	**Heme**	Tremors
Sinus sx	Abd pain	Bleeding	Syncope
Hearing loss	N/V	Bruising	**Psych**
Tinnitus	Heartburn	**Lymph**	Anxiety
Runny nose	Bloody stools	Swelling	Depression

+ ROS Findings

PE vitals **HR**   **BP**   **RR**   **T**   **SPO2**   **Ht**   **Wt**   **BMI%**

(check any)	**Neck**	**Pulm**	**Neuro**
General	( ) Midline trachea	( ) No retractions	( ) AAO x 3
( ) No Acute Distress	( ) nl thyroid w/o	( ) No dullness	( ) CN II-XII intact
( ) Cooperative	enlargement	( ) No fremitus	( ) nl sensation
( ) nl Hygiene	( ) No	( ) No wheezing/	( ) Reflexes 2+ &
Eyes	lymphadenopathy	rales/rhonchi	symmetrical
( ) nl conjunctiva	**CV**	**GI**	( ) nl memory
( ) PERRLA	( ) PMI	( ) No masses/	( ) nl speech
( ) Size___	nondisplaced	tenderness	**MSK**
( ) nl Fundus	( ) No murmur/	( ) No hep/	( ) nl tone
( ) nl Discs/vessels	gallop/rub	splenomegaly	( ) nl bulk
( ) No scleral icterus	( ) nl intensity w/o	( ) nl bowel sounds	( ) nl gait
ENT	bruit	( ) No dullness	( ) nl ROM UE
( ) No scars/masses	( ) No JVD	( ) Heme (-) stool	( ) nl ROM LE
( ) nl canals/ TM	( ) nl femoral/pedal	**GU**	L___/5 UE R___/5
( ) nl hearing bilat	pulses	( ) nl ext genitalia	L___/5 LE R___/5
( ) nl teeth/tongue	( ) No pedal	( ) No hernia	
	edema		

+ PE Findings

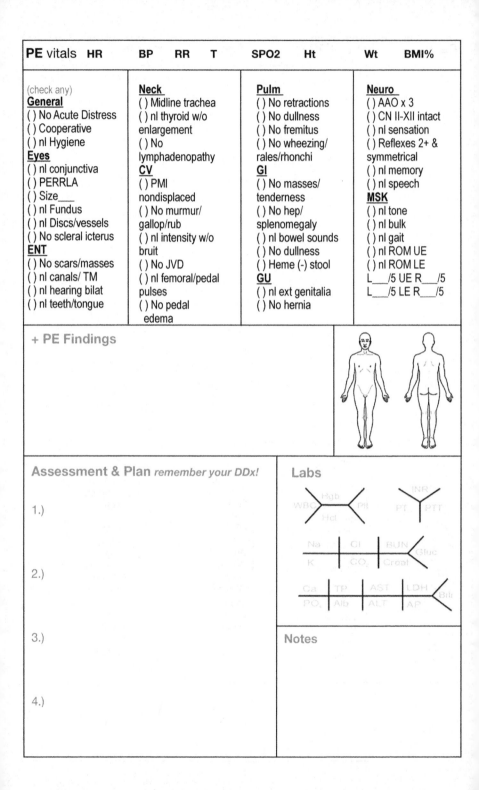

Assessment & Plan *remember your DDx!*

1.)

2.)

3.)

4.)

Labs

Notes

Date:	Initials/MRN:	Age:	Rotation:

CC: _____ y/o M/F
HPI: *symptoms/pertinent +/- ROS/prior episodes/recent travel/sick contacts*

PMHx *child/adult illness /hospitalizations/ immunizations*	**SurgHx** *type/when/ why/complications*	**FamHx** *parents/siblings/ children*

SHx *smoker/ETOH/illicits/exercise/sex/maritalstatus*

Allergies *meds/foods/ environmental/reactions*	**Meds** *reason/dose/time/route/compliance/vitamins/ herbs/otcs*

ROS (circle any)

Gen	**Pulm**	**GU**	**Endo**
Fatigue	Cough	Dysuria	Polyuria
Weight +/-	SOB	Frequency	Polydypsia
Chills	Wheezing	Hematuria	Polyphagia
Night sweats	Hemoptysis	Discharge	**Derm**
Eyes	**CV**	Flank pain	Rash
Pain	Chest pain	**MS**	Pruritis
Redness	Edema	Arthralgia	Wound(s)
Vision changes	PND	Arthritis	**Neuro**
ENT	Orthopnea	Joint swelling	Weakness
Headache	Palpitations	Myalgias	Seizures
Hoarseness	Claudication	Back pain	Parasthesias
Sore throat	**GI**	**Heme**	Tremors
Sinus sx	Abd pain	Bleeding	Syncope
Hearing loss	N/V	Bruising	**Psych**
Tinnitus	Heartburn	**Lymph**	Anxiety
Runny nose	Bloody stools	Swelling	Depression

+ ROS Findings

PE vitals   HR   BP   RR   T   SPO2   Ht   Wt   BMI%

(check any) **General**	**Neck**	**Pulm**	**Neuro**
( ) No Acute Distress	( ) Midline trachea	( ) No retractions	( ) AAO x 3
( ) Cooperative	( ) nl thyroid w/o	( ) No dullness	( ) CN II-XII intact
( ) nl Hygiene	enlargement	( ) No fremitus	( ) nl sensation
Eyes	( ) No	( ) No wheezing/	( ) Reflexes 2+ &
( ) nl conjunctiva	lymphadenopathy	rales/rhonchi	symmetrical
( ) PERRLA	**CV**	**GI**	( ) nl memory
( ) Size___	( ) PMI	( ) No masses/	( ) nl speech
( ) nl Fundus	nondisplaced	tenderness	**MSK**
( ) nl Discs/vessels	( ) No murmur/	( ) No hep/	( ) nl tone
( ) No scleral icterus	gallop/rub	splenomegaly	( ) nl bulk
ENT	( ) nl intensity w/o	( ) nl bowel sounds	( ) nl gait
( ) No scars/masses	bruit	( ) No dullness	( ) nl ROM UE
( ) nl canals/ TM	( ) No JVD	( ) Heme (-) stool	( ) nl ROM LE
( ) nl hearing bilat	( ) nl femoral/pedal	**GU**	L___/5 UE R___/5
( ) nl teeth/tongue	pulses	( ) nl ext genitalia	L___/5 LE R___/5
	( ) No pedal	( ) No hernia	
	edema		

+ PE Findings

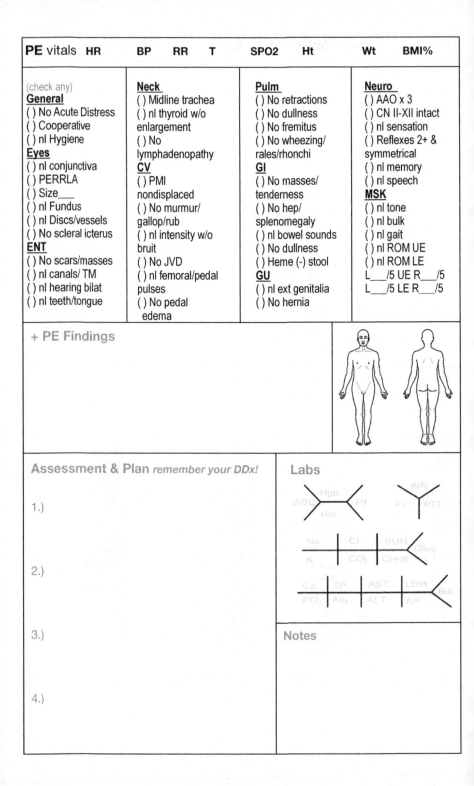

Assessment & Plan *remember your DDx!*

1.)

2.)

3.)

4.)

Labs

Notes

Date:	Initials/MRN:	Age:	Rotation:

CC: _____ y/o M/F
HPI: *symptoms/pertinent +/- ROS/prior episodes/recent travel/sick contacts*

PMHx *child/adult illness /hospitalizations/ immunizations*	**SurgHx** *type/when/ why/complications*	**FamHx** *parents/siblings/ children*

SHx *smoker/ETOH/illicits/exercise/sex/maritalstatus*

Allergies *meds/foods/ environmental/reactions*	**Meds** *reason/dose/time/route/compliance/vitamins/ herbs/otcs*

ROS (circle any)

Gen	**Pulm**	**GU**	**Endo**
Fatigue	Cough	Dysuria	Polyuria
Weight +/-	SOB	Frequency	Polydypsia
Chills	Wheezing	Hematuria	Polyphagia
Night sweats	Hemoptysis	Discharge	**Derm**
Eyes	**CV**	Flank pain	Rash
Pain	Chest pain	**MS**	Pruritis
Redness	Edema	Arthralgia	Wound(s)
Vision changes	PND	Arthritis	**Neuro**
ENT	Orthopnea	Joint swelling	Weakness
Headache	Palpitations	Myalgias	Seizures
Hoarseness	Claudication	Back pain	Parasthesias
Sore throat	**GI**	**Heme**	Tremors
Sinus sx	Abd pain	Bleeding	Syncope
Hearing loss	N/V	Bruising	**Psych**
Tinnitus	Heartburn	**Lymph**	Anxiety
Runny nose	Bloody stools	Swelling	Depression

+ ROS Findings

PE vitals	HR	BP	RR	T	SPO2	Ht	Wt	BMI%

(check any)	Neck	Pulm	Neuro
General	( ) Midline trachea	( ) No retractions	( ) AAO x 3
( ) No Acute Distress	( ) nl thyroid w/o	( ) No dullness	( ) CN II-XII intact
( ) Cooperative	enlargement	( ) No fremitus	( ) nl sensation
( ) nl Hygiene	( ) No	( ) No wheezing/	( ) Reflexes 2+ &
Eyes	lymphadenopathy	rales/rhonchi	symmetrical
( ) nl conjunctiva	**CV**	**GI**	( ) nl memory
( ) PERRLA	( ) PMI	( ) No masses/	( ) nl speech
( ) Size___	nondisplaced	tenderness	**MSK**
( ) nl Fundus	( ) No murmur/	( ) No hep/	( ) nl tone
( ) nl Discs/vessels	gallop/rub	splenomegaly	( ) nl bulk
( ) No scleral icterus	( ) nl intensity w/o	( ) nl bowel sounds	( ) nl gait
ENT	bruit	( ) No dullness	( ) nl ROM UE
( ) No scars/masses	( ) No JVD	( ) Heme (-) stool	( ) nl ROM LE
( ) nl canals/ TM	( ) nl femoral/pedal	**GU**	L___/5 UE R___/5
( ) nl hearing bilat	pulses	( ) nl ext genitalia	L___/5 LE R___/5
( ) nl teeth/tongue	( ) No pedal	( ) No hernia	
	edema		

+ PE Findings

Assessment & Plan *remember your DDx!*

1.)

2.)

3.)

4.)

Labs

Notes

Made in the USA
Columbia, SC
23 September 2024

42786849R00114